Sonia A. Schiess

Einführung von Beikost in fünf europäischen Ländern

Sonia A. Schiess

Einführung von Beikost in fünf europäischen Ländern

EU Childhood Obesity Project (CHOP)

Südwestdeutscher Verlag für Hochschulschriften

Impressum/Imprint (nur für Deutschland/only for Germany)
Bibliografische Information der Deutschen Nationalbibliothek: Die Deutsche Nationalbibliothek verzeichnet diese Publikation in der Deutschen Nationalbibliografie; detaillierte bibliografische Daten sind im Internet über http://dnb.d-nb.de abrufbar.
Alle in diesem Buch genannten Marken und Produktnamen unterliegen warenzeichen-, marken- oder patentrechtlichem Schutz bzw. sind Warenzeichen oder eingetragene Warenzeichen der jeweiligen Inhaber. Die Wiedergabe von Marken, Produktnamen, Gebrauchsnamen, Handelsnamen, Warenbezeichnungen u.s.w. in diesem Werk berechtigt auch ohne besondere Kennzeichnung nicht zu der Annahme, dass solche Namen im Sinne der Warenzeichen- und Markenschutzgesetzgebung als frei zu betrachten wären und daher von jedermann benutzt werden dürften.

Verlag: Südwestdeutscher Verlag für Hochschulschriften GmbH & Co. KG
Dudweiler Landstr. 99, 66123 Saarbrücken, Deutschland
Telefon +49 681 37 20 271-1, Telefax +49 681 37 20 271-0
Email: info@svh-verlag.de

Zugl.: München, LMU, Diss., 2011

Herstellung in Deutschland:
Schaltungsdienst Lange o.H.G., Berlin
Books on Demand GmbH, Norderstedt
Reha GmbH, Saarbrücken
Amazon Distribution GmbH, Leipzig
ISBN: 978-3-8381-2732-3

Imprint (only for USA, GB)
Bibliographic information published by the Deutsche Nationalbibliothek: The Deutsche Nationalbibliothek lists this publication in the Deutsche Nationalbibliografie; detailed bibliographic data are available in the Internet at http://dnb.d-nb.de.
Any brand names and product names mentioned in this book are subject to trademark, brand or patent protection and are trademarks or registered trademarks of their respective holders. The use of brand names, product names, common names, trade names, product descriptions etc. even without a particular marking in this works is in no way to be construed to mean that such names may be regarded as unrestricted in respect of trademark and brand protection legislation and could thus be used by anyone.

Publisher: Südwestdeutscher Verlag für Hochschulschriften GmbH & Co. KG
Dudweiler Landstr. 99, 66123 Saarbrücken, Germany
Phone +49 681 37 20 271-1, Fax +49 681 37 20 271-0
Email: info@svh-verlag.de

Printed in the U.S.A.
Printed in the U.K. by (see last page)
ISBN: 978-3-8381-2732-3

Copyright © 2011 by the author and Südwestdeutscher Verlag für Hochschulschriften GmbH & Co. KG and licensors
All rights reserved. Saarbrücken 2011

Inhaltsverzeichnis

1.	**Einleitung**	3 - 12
2.	**Publikation I**	13 - 31
	´Introduction of complementary feeding in 5 European countries´	
3.	**Publikation II**	32 - 52
	´Intake of energy providing liquids during the first year of life in five European countries´	
4.	**Manuskript I**	53 - 73
	´Introduction of potential allergenic foods in the infant´s diet´	
5.	**Manuskript II**	74 - 91
	´Introduction of complementary feeding in five European countries´	
6.	**Zusammenfassung in Deutsch**	92 - 93
7.	**Zusammenfassung in Englisch**	94 - 95
8.	**Danksagung**	96
9.	**Anhang**	
	9.1. Bestätigungen Co-Autoren	97 - 106
	9.2. Beitrag Doktorandin	107 - 109
	9.3. 3-Tage Ernährungsprotokolle (1. Tag)	110 - 111

Einleitung

In keinem anderem Lebensalter verändert sich die Ernährung so stark wie im ersten Lebensjahr. Von der reinen Muttermilch bzw. Säuglingsanfangsnahrung wechselt sie über die pürierte Beikost zur Familienkost. In diesen stoffwechselaktiven und von intensivem Wachstum geprägten Monaten kann eine frühkindliche Prägung einen sowohl kurz- wie auch langfristigen Einfluss auf die Entwicklung und die Gesundheit des Säuglings haben (1;2).

Die Ernährung des Säuglings im ersten Lebensjahr, sein Wachstum und seine Gewichtszunahme werden mit Übergewicht, Adipositas, erhöhtem Blutdruck und Diabetes in späteren Jahren in Zusammenhang gebracht (3-9). Im Jahr 1999 stellten von Kries et al. bei der Eingangsuntersuchung von Schulkindern in Bayern einen starken Zusammenhang zwischen Säuglingsernährung, Übergewicht und Adipositas fest (10). Kinder, die in den ersten Lebensmonaten Säuglingsanfangsnahrung statt Muttermilch bekamen hatten eine höhere Wahrscheinlichkeit, im Alter von fünf bis sechs Jahren an Übergewicht (12.6% vs. 9.2%) oder Adipositas (4.5% vs. 2.8%) zu leiden. Kinder, die in den ersten Lebensmonaten keine Muttermilch erhielten haben im Alter von neun bis zehn Jahren einen höheren Körperfettanteil als Kinder, die in den ersten Lebensmonaten gestillt wurden (11). In verschiedenen Studien korrelierte die Dauer der Stillzeit mit einer geringeren Adipositasprävalenz im späteren Leben (2;10;12-14).

Säuglingsanfangsnahrung hat einen etwas höheren Energiegehalt sowie einen zwei- bis dreifach höheren Eiweißanteil als Muttermilch (15;16). Einige Studien zeigen, dass Säuglinge mit Säuglingsanfangsnahrung eine durchschnittlich höhere Energie- und Eiweißzufuhr im Vergleich zu gestillten Säuglingen haben (15-18). Es wird angenommen, dass die hohe Eiweißzufuhr von Säuglingen, die mit Säuglingsanfangsnahrung gefüttert werden, ein starker Einflussfaktor auf die Entwicklung von Übergewicht und Adipositas ist (19;20). Weiterhin zeigten Säuglinge mit Säuglingsanfangsnahrung bei der Beikosteinführung keine Verringerung ihrer Milchzufuhr im Gegensatz zu gestillten Säuglingen (15).

Im EU Childhood Obesity Projekt (http://www.metabolic-programming.org), einer doppelt blind randomisierten Interventionsstudie mit über 1000 gesunden, reifgeborenen Säuglingen aus verschiedenen europäischen Ländern, wird der Zusammenhang zwischen der Eiweißzufuhr im Säuglingsalter und der Entwicklung von Wachstum und Gewicht bei

Kindern nach der Geburt bis zum Alter von 8.5 Jahren untersucht (21). Die Rekrutierung der Teilnehmer wurde in 11 Studienzentren in fünf europäischen Ländern (Belgien, Deutschland, Italien, Polen und Spanien) durchgeführt und schließt somit Teilnehmer mit unterschiedlichem kulturellem und geographischem Hindergrund ein (22). Anhand von Fragebögen und regelmäßigen Besuchen der Studienteilnehmer in die Studienzentren wurden Daten zur Gesundheitsgeschichte der Eltern und der Säuglinge, so wie sozioökonomische Daten und Ernährungsgewohnheiten erfasst. Das Studienkollektiv besteht aus einer Kontrollgruppe gestillter Kinder (welche mindestens bis zum Ende des dritten Lebensmonats gestillt wurden) sowie aus zwei randomisierten Interventionsgruppen mit Säuglingen mit Säuglingsanfangsnahrung mit unterschiedlichem Eiweissgehalt, die bis zur achten Lebenswoche auf eine der Studien-Säuglingsanfangsnahrungen umgestellt wurde (21). Der Energiegehalt der beiden Säuglingsanfangsnahrungen wurde mit dem entsprechenden Fettgehalt angeglichen. Der Kohlenhydrat- und Mikronährstoffgehalt war in beiden Studien-Säuglingsmilchnahrungen identisch.

Für eine möglichst genaue Ernährungsanamnese wurden monatliche 3-Tage Wiegeprotokolle im ersten bis neunten sowie zwölften Lebensmonat eingesetzt. Diese Ernährungserhebungsmethode, ist zwar zeitaufwendig und bedarf einer guten Kooperation der Teilnehmer, stellt aber auf der anderen Seite eine qualitative und quantitativ sehr aussagekräftige Methode dar (23).

Innerhalb des EU Childhood Obestiy Projektes wurde der Frage nachgegangen, ob der unterschiedliche Eiweißgehalt in den Säuglingsanfangsnahrungen Einfluss auf den zeitlichen Beginn der Beikosteinführung, die verzehrte Nahrungsmenge sowie die Nährstoffzufuhr über die Beikost hat.

In Studien wurden, vermutlich durch die höhere Eiweißzufuhr der Säuglingsanfangsnahrung ausgelöste, erhöhte Insulinwerte beobachtet (1). Hieraus ergab sich die Frage, ob erhöhte Insulinwerte zu einem gesteigerten Hungergefühl und somit zu einer verfrühten Beikosteinführung bzw. einer vermehrten Beikostzufuhr führen.

Zunächst wurde anhand der Daten der 3-Tage Wiegeprotokolle, der Zeitpunkt der Beikosteinführung bei gestillten Säuglingen im Vergleich zu nicht gestillten Säuglingen ermittelt (24). Die WHO empfiehlt sechs Monate ausschließliches Stillen mit anschließender Beikosteinführung und einer weiterführenden Stilldauer bis zum Alter von

2 Jahren (25). In vielen europäischen Ländern wurde diese Empfehlung bis heute nicht offiziell übernommen. Die ESPGHAN (European Society for Paediatric Gastroenterology, Hepatology and Nutrition) empfiehlt eine möglichst ausschließliche Stillzeit von vier bis sechs Monaten mit einer schrittweise beginnenden Beikosteinführung (26). Beikost sollte nicht vor dem Alter von 17 Wochen und nicht nach einem Alter von 26 Wochen eingeführt werden. Diese Empfehlungen zur Beikosteinführung gelten sowohl für gestillte Säuglinge wie auch für Säuglinge, die mit Säuglingsanfangsnahrung ernährt werden. Innerhalb der Studie waren die aktuellen, offiziellen Landesempfehlungen mit einer möglichst ausschließlichen Stillzeit von 4 bis 6 Monaten und einer anschließenden Beikosteinführung zwischen den einzelnen Ländern recht ähnlich.

Wie verschiedene Studien zeigen, wird bei Säuglingen, die mit Säuglingsanfangsnahrung ernährt werden, generell früher mit der Zufütterung von Beikost angefangen als bei gestillten Säuglingen (27;28). Weitere Faktoren, die mit einer früheren Beikosteinführung in Verbindung gesetzt werden, sind ein niedrigeres Ausbildungsniveau und ein niedrigerer sozioökonomischer Status der Mutter, ein geringeres Alter der Mutter und ihre Rauchgewohnheiten (28-31).

Weiterhin war es von Interesse, den Verzehr von energiehaltigen Flüssigkeiten bei Säuglingen zu untersuchen. Laut WHO ist Muttermilch das einzige adäquate Nahrungsmittel für Säuglinge während der ersten sechs Lebensmonate, auch die ESPGHAN empfiehlt eine möglichst ausschließliche Stillzeit in den ersten vier bis sechs Lebensmonaten. Nach heutigen Erkenntnissen benötigen gesunde Säuglinge in den ersten Monaten keine weitere Flüssigkeitszufuhr neben Muttermilch oder Säuglingsanfangsnahrung (25;26). Zusätzliche Getränke bergen die Gefahr, die Zufuhr von Muttermilch oder Säuglingsmilchnahrung zu reduzieren (32-34), dazu gehören Wasser oder einfache Teeaufgüsse oft nicht zu den bevorzugten Flüssigkeiten, die an Säuglinge verabreicht werden (34). Die Zufuhr von energiehaltigen Getränken wie Säften, Instant-Tees oder süßen Erfrischungsgetränken (Limonaden, Cola) können die Entwicklung von Übergewicht und Adipositas, Diabetes, Karies, aber auch eine ungenügende Kalziumzufuhr im Kindes- und Jugendalter fördern (32;35-40). Die Geschmacksempfindungen werden schon beim Fetus und Säugling geprägt, und praktizierte Ernährungsgewohnheiten in jungen Jahren haben einen bleibenden Einfluss auf den weiteren Lebensstil bis ins Alter (41). Somit gingen wir innerhalb des EU Childhood Obesity Projekt der Frage nach, inwieweit Säuglinge schon in ihren ersten Lebensmonaten energiehaltige Flüssigkeiten (Instant-Tees, Obst- und Gemüsesäfte oder süße Erfrischungsgetränke) erhalten.

Eine wachsende Herausforderung in der Pädiatrie sind die zunehmenden Nahrungsmittelallergien im Säuglings- und Kindesalter. Ca. 6 % der Säuglinge und Kleinkinder leiden unter Nahrungsmittelallergien (42). Der Zeitpunkt der Beikosteinführung scheint eine wichtige Rolle in der Allergieentwicklung zu haben, Säuglinge mit frühzeitiger Beikosteinführung (vor dem vierten Lebensmonat) zeigten ein gehäuftes Auftreten von atopischen Erkrankungen (43-46). Weiterhin hat die Auswahl der Nahrungsmittel vermutlich einen Einfluss auf die Entwicklung von akuten und chronisch allergischen Reaktionen (47). Somit wurde, unter Berücksichtigung der teilweise unterschiedlichen Landesempfehlungen, der Zeitpunkt der Einführung von potentiell allergenen Nahrungsmitteln bei gestillten und nicht gestillten Säuglingen untersucht. Aktuelle Erkenntnisse haben zu vereinfachten Empfehlungen zur Einführung von potentiell allergenen Nahrungsmitteln geführt (48). Diese Empfehlungen wurden in der Datenauswertung nicht berücksichtigt, da die vorliegende Datenerhebung zu einem früheren Zeitpunkt stattfand.

Resultate und Schlussfolgerungen

Ein erheblicher Anteil der Säuglinge erhielt schon vor Ende des vierten Lebensmonats Beikost. Obwohl für gestillte Säuglinge wie auch für nicht gestillte Säuglinge die gleichen Empfehlungen zur Beikosteinführung galten, wurde bei Säuglingen mit Säuglingsmilchnahrung ein früherer Verzehr von Beikost beobachtet. Am Ende des dritten und vierten Monats, hatten schon 6% bzw. 37.2% der Säuglinge, die mit Säuglingsmilchnahrung gefüttert wurden, im Gegensatz dazu aber nur 0.6% bzw. 17.3% der gestillten Säuglinge Beikost erhalten. Die unterschiedliche Nährstoffzusammensetzung der Studiensäuglingsmilch hatte keinen wesentlichen Einfluss auf den Zeitpunkt der Beikosteinführung. Allerdings war der Zeitpunkt der Beikosteinführung zwischen den verschiedenen Ländern signifikant unterschiedlich. Nach Anpassung eines multiplen Regressions-Modells mit Aufnahme der Variablen `Alter der Mutter´, `Ausbildungsniveau der Mutter´ und `Wohnsitz der Eltern´ fanden sich signifikante Unterschiede zwischen den Ländern. Im Vergleich zu Deutschland fand sich in Belgien bei Säuglingen, die mit Säuglingsanfangsnahrung ernährt wurden am Ende des dritten und vierten Monats ein drei- bis vierfach erhöhtes Risiko Beikost einzuführen. Bei den gestillten Säuglingen fand sich am Ende des vierten Monats sogar ein 16-fach höheres Risiko in Belgien und ein siebenfach höheres Risiko in Spanien als in Deutschland, Beikost einzuführen. Weiterhin hatten Faktoren wie das Alter der Mutter, ein niedrigeres Bildungsniveau als auch das

Rauchen einen signifikanten Einfluss auf den Zeitpunkt der Beikosteinführung. Die nationalen Empfehlungen der teilnehmenden Länder zur zeitlichen Beikosteinführung sind sehr ähnlich. Wir vermuten auf Grund unserer Resultate einen starken kulturellen und individuellen Einfluss auf die Praxis der Beikostfütterung.

Bei einem hohen Anteil von Säuglingen mit Säuglingsanfangsnahrung wurden schon ab dem ersten Monat energiehaltige Flüssigkeiten verabreicht. Nicht gestillte Säuglinge erhielten signifikant früher und in einem signifikant höheren Prozentsatz energiehaltige Getränke als gestillte Säuglinge (entsprechend 43 % und 13 % am Ende des vierten Monats). Anhand einer multiplen Regressions-Analyse mit den Einflussfaktoren `Alter der Mutter´, `Ausbildungsniveau der Mutter´ und `Wohnsitz der Eltern´ zeigte sich das Herkunftsland als ein beständiger Risikofaktor für eine frühere Einführung von energiehaltigen Flüssigkeiten bei gestillten und nicht gestillten Säuglingen.
In Polen fand sich der höchste Anteil von Säuglingen, die energiehaltige Flüssigkeiten erhielten - vor allem bei den Säuglingen mit Säuglingsanfangsnahrung - und in Belgien und Italien fand sich der niedrigste Anteil von Säuglingen, die energiehaltige Flüssigkeiten erhielten. Es gab keinen wesentlichen Unterschied im Konsumverhalten von energiehaltigen Flüssigkeiten zwischen beiden Gruppen mit Säuglingsanfangsnahrung.
Bemerkenswert war ein signifikanter Einfluss des Verzehrs von energiehaltigen Flüssigkeiten auf eine geringere Aufnahme von Flaschenmilch im Alter von zwei, drei, vier und fünf Monaten, sowie auch eine signifikant geringere Beikostzufuhr im Alter von sieben, acht, neun und zwölf Monaten. Die Säuglinge verzehrten in den ersten Monaten bevorzugt Instant-Tee und im zweiten Lebenshalbjahr Fruchtsäfte. Dabei sollte beachtet werden, dass energiehaltige Flüssigkeiten vorzugsweise Kohlenhydratlieferanten sind und wenn sie anstatt von Muttermilch oder Säuglingsanfangsnahrung getrunken werden wichtige Nährstoffe verdrängen, die für die Entwicklung und das Wachstum des Säuglings von großer Wichtigkeit sind.

Potentiell allergene Nahrungsmittel wurden signifikant früher bei Säuglingen mit Säuglingsanfangsnahrung eingeführt als bei gestillten Säuglingen. Im Alter von 4 Monaten verzehrten 6 % der gestillten und 13 % der nicht gestillten Säuglinge potentiell allergene Nahrungsmittel. Eine Ausnahme war der Verzehr von Sojaeiweiß. Im Vergleich zu nicht gestillten Säuglingen erhielten die gestillten Säuglinge zu einem signifikant früheren Zeitpunkt und zu einem signifikant höheren Anteil Sojaeiweiß.

Ebenfalls zu beobachten war ein signifikanter Unterschied im Zeitpunkt der Einführung von potentiell allergenen Nahrungsmitteln zwischen den Ländern. Nach Anpassung eines multiplen Regressions-Models mit Aufnahme der Variablen `Alter der Mutter´, `Ausbildungsniveau der Mutter´, `Rauchgewohnheiten der Mutter´, `Allergien bei der Mutter´ und `Wohnsitz der Eltern´ zeigte sich das Herkunftsland als konsistenter und signifikanter Einflussfaktor.

Zusammenfassend konnte beobachtet werden, dass trotz gleicher Empfehlungen nicht gestillte Säuglinge zu einem signifikant früheren Zeitpunkt und zu signifikanten höheren Anteilen feste Beikost, energiehaltige Getränke wie auch potentiell allergene Nahrungsmittel erhielten. Weiterhin fanden sich trotz ähnlicher Empfehlungen signifikante Unterschiede zwischen den Ländern im Bezug auf die zeitliche Einführung von Beikost, ob als feste Nahrungsmittel, energiehaltige Getränke oder als potentiell allergene Nahrungsmittel, bei den gestillten sowie nicht gestillten Säuglingen. Die unterschiedliche Nährstoffzusammensetzung der Studien-Säuglingsanfangsnahrung hatte keinen Einfluss auf das Alter der Beikosteinführung. Die Zufuhr von energiehaltigen Getränken wirkte sich signifikant auf eine geringere Aufnahme von Säuglingsanfangsnahrung in den ersten Lebensmonaten aus sowie auf eine signifikant geringere Beikostzufuhr im Alter von sieben, acht, neun und zwölf Monaten. Die Ernährung des Säuglings in seinen ersten Monaten, wie auch seine kulturellen und geographischen Hintergründe zeigten einen signifikanten Einfluss auf das Alter der Beikosteinführung. Weiterhin hatten der Ausbildungsgrad der Mutter, das Alter der Mutter wie auch ihre Rauchgewohnheiten signifikante Einflüsse auf den Zeitpunkt der Beikosteinführung. Eine gute Information und Aufklärung wie auch Begleitung an die Eltern, speziell von Säuglingen, die Säuglingsanfangsnahrung erhalten, über die zeitlich korrekte Einführung der Beikost, in fester und flüssiger Form wäre sehr wünschenswert.

Reference List

1. Koletzko B, von Kries R, Monasterolo RC et al. Can infant feeding choices modulate later obesity risk? Am J Clin Nutr 2009;89(5):S1502-S1508.
2. Owen CG, Martin RM, Whincup PH, Smith GD, Cook DG. Effect of Infant Feeding on the Risk of Obesity Across the Life Course: A Quantitative Review of Published Evidence. Pediatrics 2005;115:1367-77.
3. Lucas A, Fewtrell MS, Cole TJ. Fetal origins of adult disease---the hypothesis revisited. BMJ 1999;319:245-9.
4. Toschke AM, Grote V, Koletzko B, von Kries R. Identifying children at high risk for overweight at school entry by weight gain during the first 2 years. Arch Pediat Adolesc Med 2004;158(5):449-52.
5. Arenz S, Rückelr R, Koletzko B, von Kries R. Breast-feeding and childhood obesity - a systematic review. Int J Obes 2004;28:1247-56.
6. Scaglioni S, Agostini C, Notaris R et al. Early macronutrient intake and overweight at five years of age. Int J Obes Relat Metab Disord 2007;24(6):777-81.
7. Singhal A, Lanigan JA. Breastfeeding. early growth and later obesity. Pediatr Allergy Immunol 2007;8(Suppl.1):51-4.
8. Singhal A, Cole TJ, Lucas A. Early nutrition in preterm infants and later blood pressure: two cohorts after randomised trials. Lancet 2001;357:413-9.
9. Owen CG, Martin RM, Whincup PH, Smith GD, Cook DG. Does breastfeeding influence risk of type 2 diabetes in later life? A quantitative analysis of published evidence. Am J Clin Nutr 2006;84:1043-54.
10. von Kries R, Koletzko B, Sauerwald T et al. Breast feeding and obesity: cross sectional study. BMJ 1999;319:147-50.
11. Toschke AM, Vignerova J, Lhotska L, Osancova K, Koletzko B, von Kries R. Overweight and obesity in 6- to 14-year-old Czech children in 1991: Protective effect of breast-feeding. J Pediatr 2002;141:764-9.
12. Schack-Nielsen L, Michaelsen KF, Mortensen EL, Sørensen TIA, Reinisch JM. Protecting infants through human milk: Is duration of breastfeeding influencing the risk of obesity in adult males ? Adv Exp Med Biol 2004;554:383-5.
13. Harder T, Bergmann R, Kallischnigg G, Plagemann A. Duration of Breastfeeding and Risk of Overweight: A Meta-Analysis. Am J Epidemiol 2005;162:397-403.
14. Grummer-Strawn LM, Mei Z. Does Breastfeeding Protect Against Pediatric Overweight? Analysis of Longitudinal Data From the Centers for Disease Control and Prevention Pediatric Nutrition Surveillance System. Pediatrics 2004;113:e81-e86.

15. Heinig MJ, Nommsen LA, Peerson JM, Lonnerdal B, Dewey KG. Energy and protein intakes of breast-fed and formula-fed infants during the first year of life and their association with growth velocity: the DARLING Study. Am J Clin Nutr 1993;58:152-61.

16. Alexy U, Kersting M, Sichert-Hellert W, Manz F, Schöch G. Macronutrient Intake of 3- to 36-Month-Old German Infants and Children: Results of the DONALD Study. Ann Nutr Metab 1999;43:14-22.

17. De Bruin NC, Degenhart HJ, Gal S, Westerterp KR, Stijnen T, Visser HK. Energy utilization and growth in breast-fed and formula-fed infants measured prospectively during the first year of life. Am J Clin Nutr 1998;67:885-96.

18. Butte NF, Wong WW, Hopkinson JM, Smith EO, Ellis KJ. Infant Feeding Mode Affects Early Growth and Body Composition. Pediatrics 2000;106:1355-66.

19. Rolland-Cachera MF, Deheeger M, Bellisle F, Sempe M, Guilloud-Bataille M, Patois E. Adiposity rebound in children: a simple indicator for predicting obesity. Am J Clin Nutr 1984;39:129-35.

20. Koletzko B. Long-term consequences of early feeding on later obesity risk. In: Protein and Energy Requirements in Infancy and Childhood. Rigo J, Ziegler E. eds. Nestlec Ltd, Karger Publishing. 2006:1-18.

21. Koletzko B, von Kries R, Monasterolo RC et al. Lower protein in infant formula is associated with lower weight up to age 2 y: a randomized clinical trial. Am J Clin Nutr 2009;89:1-10.

22. Naska A, Fouskakis D, Oikonomou E et al. Dietary patterns and their socio-demographic determinants in 10 European countries: data from the DAFNE databank. Eur J Clin Nutr 2005;60:181-90.

23. Schneider R. Welche Methoden gibt es, Ernährungsinfomationen zu ermitteln. S.101-127. In: Vom Umgang mit Zahlen und Daten. Umschau Zeitschriftenverlag, Frankfurt am Main 1997.

24. Schiess, S., Grote, V., Scaglioni, S, Luque, V., Martin, F., Stolarczyk, A, Vechi, F., and Koletzko, B. Introduction of complementary feeding in five European countries. J Pediatr Gastroenterol Nutr 50(1), 92-98.

25. WHO 54th World Health Assembly. Infant and young child nutrition. WHA54.2. Ref Type: Report.

26. ESPGHAN Committee of Nutrition: Agostoni C, Decsi T, Fewtrell M et al. Complementary feeding: a commentary by the ESPGHAN Committee on Nutrition. J Pediatr Gastroenterol Nutr 2008;46:99-110.

27. Noble S, Emmett P. Differences in weaning practice, food and nutrient intake between breast- and formula-fed 4-month-old infants in England. J Hum Nutr Dietet 2006;19:303-13.

28. Fewtrell M, Lucas A, Morgan J. Factors associated with the age of introduction of solid foods in full and preterm infants. Arch Dis Child 2003;88:F296-F301.

29. Fein SB, Labiner-Wolfe J, Scanlon KS, Grummer-Strawn LM. Selected Complementary Feeding Practices and Their Association With Maternal Education. Pediatrics 2008;122:S91-S97.

30. Lanigan JA, Bishop JA, Kimber AC, Morgan J. Review: Systemic review concerning the age of introduction of complementary foods to the healthy full-term infant. Eur J Clin Nutr 2001;55:309-20.

31. Alder EM, Williams FL, Anderson AS, Forsyth S, Florey C, van der Velde P. What influence the timing of the introduction of solid food to infants ? Brit J Nutr 2004;92(3):527-31.

32. AAP Committee on Nutrition. The Use and Misuse of Fruit Juice in Pediatrics. Pediatrics 2001;107:1210-3.

33. Marshall TLS, Broffitt B, Eichenberger-Gilmore J, Stumbo J. Beverage consumption and infant nutrition - Benefits of milk vs. juice. Nutrition Research Newsletter 2003.

34. Emmett, P., North, K., Noble, S., and ALSPAC Study Team. Types of drinks consumed by infants at 4 and 8 months of age: a descriptive study. Public Health Nutrition 3(2), 211-217.

35. Malik VS, Schulze MB, Hu FB. Intake of sugar-sweetened beverages and weight gain: a systematic review. Am J Clin Nutr 2006;84:274-88.

36. Ludwig DS, Peterson KE, Gortmaker SL. Relation between consumption of sugar-sweetened drinks and childhood obesity: a prospective, observational analysis. Lancet 2001;357:505-8.

37. Vartanian LR, Schwartz MB, Brownell KD. Effects of soft drink consumption on nutrition and health: a systematic review and meta-analysis. Am J Public Health 2007;97(4):667-75.

38. Faith MS, Dennison BA, Edmunds LS, Stratton HH. Fruit Juice Intake Predicts Increased Adiposity Gain in Children From Low-Income Families: Weight Status-by-Environment Interaction. Pediatrics 2006;118:2066-75.

39. Saalfield S, Jackson-Allen P. Biopsychosocial consequences of sweetened drink consumption in children 0-6 years of age. Pediatric Nursing 2006;32(5):460-71.

40. Forschungsinstitut für Kinderernährung. Erfrischungsgetränke und Ernährungsqualität. Ernährungs-Umschau 2008;11:646.

41. Ellrott, T. Wie Kinder essen lernen. Ernährung 2007: 167-173.

42. Poole JA, Barriga K, Leung DYM et al. Timing of Initial Exposure to Cereal Grains and the Risk of Wheat Allergy. Pediatrics 2006;117:2175-82.

43. Fergusson DM, Horwood LJ, Shannon FT. Early Solid Feeding and Recurrent Childhood Eczema: A 10-Year Longitudinal Study. Pediatrics 1990;86:541-6.

44. Muraro A, Dreborg S, Halken S et al. Dietary prevention of allergic diseases in infants and small children. Part III: Critical review of published peer-reviewed observational

and interventional studies and final recommendations. Pediatr Allergy Immunol 2004;15:291-307.

45. Wilson AC, Forsyth JS, Greene SA, Irvine L, Hau C, Howie PW. Relation of infant diet to childhood health: seven year follow up of cohort of children in Dundee infant feeding study. BMJ 1998;316:21-5.

46. Oddy WH, Holt PG, Sly PD et al. Association between breast feeding and asthma in 6 year old children: findings of a prospective birth cohort study. BMJ 1999;319:815-9.

47. Fergusson DM, Horwood LJ. Early solid food diet and eczema in childhood: a 10-year longitudinal study. Pediatr Allergy Immunol 1994;5(Suppl):44-7.

48. Greer FR, Sicherer SH, Burks AW, and the Committee on Nutrition and Section on Allergy and Immunology. Effects of Early Nutritional Interventions on the Development of Atopic Disease in Infants and Children: The Role of Maternal Dietary Restriction, Breastfeeding, Timing of Introduction of Complementary Foods, and Hydrolyzed Formulas. Pediatrics 2008;121:183-91.

Introduction of complementary feeding in five European countries

Sonia Schiess[1] Mag Human Nutr, Veit Grote[2] MD MSc, Silvia Scaglioni[3] MD, Verónica Luque[4] Nutritionist, Francoise Martin[5] Nutritionist, Anna Stolarczyk[6] Ph.D. Nutritionist, Fiammetta Vecchi[3] B Sc, Berthold Koletzko[1] MD PhD Prof., for the European Childhood Obesity Project *

[1]Div. Metabolic Diseases & Nutritional Medicine, Dr. von Hauner Children's Hospital, Ludwig-Maximilian University, Germany, [2] Dept. Epidemiology, Inst. of Social Pediatrics and Adolescent Medicine, Ludwig-Maximilian University, Germany [3]Dept. of Pediatrics, San Paolo Hospital, Milan, Italy, [4]Dept. of Medicine & Surgery Pediatrics Unit, University Rovira i Virgili, Reus, Spain, [5]CHC St. Vincent, Rocourt, Belgium, [6]Clinic of Pediatrics, Children's Memorial Health Institute, Warsaw, Poland

*Study team:

Belgium (ULB Bruxelles and CHC St Vincent Liège): Carlier C, Goyens P, Hoyos J, Langhendries J-P, Martin F, Van Hees J-N, Xhonneux A **Germany** (Division of Nutritional Medicine and Metabolism, Dr. von Hauner Children's Hospital, and Division of Pediatric Epidemiology, Institute of Social Pediatrics and Adolescent Medicine, Ludwig Maximilians University of Munich): Beyer J, Demmelmair H, Fritsch M, Handel U, Hannibal I, Kreichauf S, von Kries R, Pawellek I, Verwied-Jorky S **Italy** (University of Milan): Giovannini M, Agostoni C, Confalonieri F, Scaglioni S, Tedeschi S, Vecchi F, Verduci E **Spain** (Universitat Rovira i Virgili): Closa Monasterolo R, Escribano Subias J, Méndez Riera G, Luque Moreno V **Poland** (Children's Memorial Health Institute): Socha J, Dobrzańska A, Gruszfeld D, Socha P, Stolarczyk A, Janas R, Pietraszek E, Kowalik A

Publihed in Journal of Pediatric Gastroenterology & Nutrition. 50(1):92-98, Jan 2010

Abstract

Objectives: Little is known on the practice of introducing complementary feeding across Europe. We aim at describing times of solid introduction in healthy infants in five European countries.

Methods: Between October 2002 and June 2004, 1678 healthy term infants fed either breast milk (BF) for at least 4 months (n=588) or study formula (FF) (n=1090) with different protein contents were included. Three-day-weighed food protocols were obtained at ages 1, 2, 3, 4, 5, 6, 7, 8, 9 and 12 completed months.

Results: Solids were introduced earlier in FF infants (median: 19 weeks, IQR: 17-21) than BF infants (median: 21 weeks, IQR: 19-24). Some 37.2% of FF infants and 17.2 % of BF infants received solid foods at 4 completed months and hence earlier than recommended in Europe. Solids had been introduced at 7 completed months in 99.3% of FF infants and 97.7% of BF infants, respectively. Belgium had the highest percentage of solid feeding in FF infants at 3 (15.8%) and 4 (55.6%) completed months, and in BF infants at 4 (43%) and 5 (84.8%) completed months. Multiple regression showed low maternal age, low education level, and maternal smoking to predictors an early introduction of solids at 3 and 4 completed months.

Conclusions: Complementary feeding is introduced earlier than recommended in a sizeable number of infants, particularly among formula fed infants. Country and population specific approaches to adequately inform parents should be explored.

Introduction

Healthy infants should receive complementary feeding from the end of the first half year of life, when breast feeding or infant formula alone cannot always secure an adequate nutrient supply. Since 2001, the World Health Organisation (WHO) recommendation is to introduce complementary foods from the seventh month of life, rather than in the 5th or 6th month as previously recommended (1;2). While the WHO recommendation addresses all countries, advisory bodies in industrialized countries continue to recommend an age range for introduction of complementary foods. The European Society of Paediatric Gastroenterology, Hepatology and Nutrition (ESPGHAN) supports exclusive or full breast-feeding for about 6 months as a desirable goal and recommends to introduce complementary feeding not before 17 weeks and not later than 26 weeks (3). The American Academy of Pediatrics recommends that solid foods should not be introduced before 4 to 6 months of age (4).

In Germany the recommendation at the time of recruitment was exclusive breastfeeding for the first 4 to 6 months with the introduction of Beikost from the age of 5 to 7 months (5) (6), (Nationale Stillkommission: http://www.bfr.bund.de/cd/922). In Belgium recommendations of the O.N.E. (L´Office de la Naissance et de l´Enfance), an institution that supports and assesses the well-being of children from 0 to 12 months outside of his or her family, are not to start with the introduction of complementary feeding before the age of 4 completed months (7). In Italy, the Italian Society of Neonatology (SIN) recommended in 2002 that in term, healthy babies can continue breastfeeding exclusively for 6 months, whereas introduction of complementary foods can be started with 4 or 5 months depending on maternal and infant circumstances (8). In Poland as well as in Spain recommendations state that complementary feeding should not start before 4 completed months of age (9-11).

Cultural and socio-demographic characteristics of families may influence infant feeding patterns. In some studies earlier introduction of complementary foods were found associated with lower socioeconomics status (12-14) and education level (15;16), maternal smoking (16) and younger age of the mother (15;17). In some studies formula fed infants started complementary foods earlier than breast fed infants (12;13;15;17).

We analyzed data of food protocols from five European countries with similar infant feeding recommendations, which were collected as part of the prospective European Childhood Obesity Project, with the aim to explore whether type of milk feeding, country of residence or other factors were associated with the introduction of solids.

Materials and Methods
Study Design
The data evaluated was collected as part of the European **Ch**ildhood **O**besity **P**roject (CHOP), a multicentre intervention trial in 5 European countries to investigate the relation of the infant diet and protein supply on early growth and later obesity risk (18).

Eligible for study participation were apparently healthy, singleton, term infants who were born between 1st October 2002 and 31st July 2004 in Germany (Munich and Nuremberg), Belgium (Brussels and Liège), Italy (Milano), Spain (Tarragona and Reus) and Poland (Warsaw). Mothers were approached by trained study personnel in maternity hospitals before their discharge or contacted via midwifes or paediatricians. Infants were enrolled during the first 8 weeks of life. Excluded were mothers with a hormonal or metabolic disease (e.g. gestational diabetes) or intake of drugs during pregnancy that are known to influence infants growth (e.g. thyroid hormones, anti thyroid drugs, Corticosteroids). Moving too far away from the study centre to come for visits was a further reason for exclusion.

Dietary intervention, study formulas
Study groups included a breastfed reference group (BF) and 2 groups of infants fed study formula with exclusive formula feeding (FF) starting between birth and the age of week 8, which were randomized to one of our study formulas with either higher and lower protein content. Infant formulas had a protein content of 7.1% and 11.7% of energy (1.25g protein /100ml and 2.1g protein/100ml) and follow on formulas 8.8% and 17.6% of energy (1.6g protein/100ml and 3.2g protein/100ml) for the lower and higher protein group, respectively. Equal energy content was achieved by adapting fat content, while the intake of carbohydrates and other nutrients was not different (18). The study formulas were provided by Bledina, Steenvorde, France and supplied to families until the infant age of 1 year.

There was no further intervention addressing infant dietary intakes. Information on dietary intakes of infants were collected prospectively with a 3-day-weighed food records, which included 2 week days and 1 weekend day, at the age of each completed month from 1 to 9 months, and at 12 completed months. The 3-day food protocol collected information on all dietary intakes of the infant, including breast milk, formula, and any other liquids or foods. The regular study visits and additional contacts by mailings and phone calls between study personnel and parents allowed to clarify arising questions on filling out the dietary protocol, and to enhance compliance. Mothers/parents were provided with a study telephone hotline number for more information and to address any arising questions.

Data procedure

Dietary food records were checked by nutritionists at each study centre; to clarify any questions parents were contacted if necessary; data were then introduced to the specifically developed nutrition software "NutrCalc" and transferred to a central data base. Standard Operating Procedures (SOPs) were developed to harmonize the introduction of food intake data and the calculations of dieticians in the different study centres.

Complementary foods

Complementary food items were categorized as food groups and according to their ingredients. For our analysis solids included food items such as beef, cereals or bread, egg, fat, fish, fruit, meat, milk or milk products, nuts or seeds, potatoes, poultry, pulses, sausages, soy or soy products, sweets or infant sweets and vegetables. Each food item was classified either as a commercial infant product (CIP) if it was offered as baby food for the first year of life (excluding infant or follow-on formula), or as normal food (NF) offered for consumption not only by infants but also by children or adults.

Socio-demographic data

We grouped mothers in four categories based on age at birth: I= ≤25 years, II= >25 to 30 years, III= >30 to 35 years and IV= >35 years. Maternal educational levels were categorised in 3 groups: *no/low* =pre-preliminary to lower secondary, *middle* = upper secondary and post-secondary non-tertiary and *high* = first and second stage of tertiary education according to standard ISCED (International Standard Classification of Education).

Dropouts

For the formula group 1090 infants were enrolled, of whom 851 participated in the follow-up visits at 6 months and 767 at 12 months; for the observational group of breast fed infants 588 infants were enrolled, of whom 349 participated in the follow-up visits at 6 months, 327 at 12 months. Thus, 687 infants dropped out until the age of 12 month for the following reasons: refusal of parents/loss of contact (310/45%), no compliance with assigned milk feeding (250/36%), address unknown (51/7%), moving out of the study region (27/4%), exclusion of illness/medication (12/2%) and other reason/unknown (37/5%).

Statistics

Stata 9.2, SPSS 16.0, and Excel were used for data analyses. Chi square and multiple logistic regression analysis were used to adjust differences in solid introduction at each month by confounders.

Ethics

The study was approved by the ethics committees of all study centres. Written informed parental consent was obtained for each infant.

Results

A total of 1678 infants were enrolled (1090 FF infants and 588 BF infants, 65% and 35% respectively) into the study. For 1366 (81.4%) infants (928 FF infants and 438 BF infants, 68% and 32% respectively) at least one iterative 3 day-food protocol could be evaluated (**Table 1**). At the age of 1 month some 1045 three-day-food protocols were evaluated, at 2 months 1208, at 3 months 1184, at 4 months 1136, at 5 months 1128, at 6 months 1075, at 7 months 1008, at 8 months 984, at 9 months 967 and at 12 months 945 three-day-food protocols.

The socio-demographic characteristics of study participants are shown in **Table 1**. Except for country we did not find differences in socio demographic characteristics of those infants with food protocols and those without protocols. However, the proportion of filled-in protocols varied between countries (p<0.001), with a lower participation rate in Belgium and a higher participation rate in Italy. Since the socio-demographic characteristics of our FF and BF infants differed in many aspects, we separated both groups in the analysis.

Solids had been introduced in 6% of FF infants at the age of 3 completed months, in 37.2% at 4, 96.2% at 6 and 99.3% at 7 completed months, respectively (**Figure 1**). The median age of introduction was 19 weeks (IQR: 17-21). Among the BF infants only 0.6% had received solids at the age of 3 completed months, whereas 17.3%, 87.1% and 97.7% received solids at the ages of 4, 6 and 7 months, respectively, with a median age at introduction of 21 weeks (IQR: 19-24) (**Figure 1**).

A higher proportion of FF infants received commercial infant products (CIP) than normal foods (NF) during the first year of life. In contrast, fewer breast fed infants consumed CIP than NF (**Table 2**).

FF infants

There were significant differences between countries in the time point of introduction of solids during the first 8 months of life (**Table 3**). We found an early introduction of solids in Belgium, with 15.8% and 55.6% at the ages of 3 and 4 completed months, respectively. At the age of 3 completed months, Italy and Poland had the lowest proportion of FF infants receiving solids with only 2.4% and 3.1%, respectively. In all countries at the age of 6

completed months more than 90% of FF infants received some solids.

Younger mothers (≤ 25 years) of formula fed infants introduced solids significantly earlier during the first 4 months of life to their infant's diet (at 1, 3 and 4 completed months: $p<0.05$). Logistic regression showed a 2.9 fold higher probability that younger mothers ($\leq$

25 years) start to introduce solids at the age of 3 months than mothers older than 35 years. A low maternal education had a 1.8 higher risk and maternal smoking 3 months prior and during early pregnancy had a 1.5 higher risk to introduce some solids at the age of 4 months.

Applying multiple regression analysis including the effects of maternal age, education level, smoking behaviour and country of residence on the introduction of solids in FF infants, we found a 4 fold higher probability for introduction of solids at the age of 3 completed months in Belgian FF infants (OR=3.96), and a 3 fold higher risk (OR=2.86) in the youngest group of mothers ($\leq$ 25 years).

The probability to have solids introduced already at the age of 4 completed months was 3 fold higher in Belgium (OR=3.28), 2 fold higher for low maternal educational level (OR=1.87) and 1.4 fold higher for mothers who smoked (OR=1.40) (**Table 4**).

The different protein and fat levels of the study formulas did not influence the time of introducing solids. Neither was the birth weight, birth order or gender of the FF infants related to the time point of introduction of any solid.

BF infants

Between the age of 4 and 6 completed months, introduction of solids differed significantly by country. Up to 3 completed months, solids were not given to more than 1.4% of BF infants in any country. At the age of 4 and 5 completed months Belgium had the highest proportion (43.2% and 84.8%), and Germany (4.9% and 25.0%) and Poland (6.7% and 36.2%) the lowest proportion of BF infants receiving solids.

At 6 completed months of age at least 84% of BF infants in every country received some solids except in Germany (69.5%), and at 7 completed months more than 93% of all BF infants in each country had solids introduced (**Table 5**).

Low maternal education level was significantly associated with the introduction of solids at 3 and 4 completed months (3 months: $p<0.001$, 4 months: $p<0.05$) in univariate analysis, while multiple regression analysis showed an effect only at 4 months. Maternal age and smoking behaviour was unrelated to timing of introduction of solids.

Applying multiple regression analysis, including the effects of maternal age, education level, smoking behaviour and country of residence, receiving solids at 4 completed months was 16 times more likely (OR=15.93) in Belgium and 7 times more likely in Spain (OR=6.60) compared to German BF infants. Low- and middle-level maternal education had a 3 fold higher association (OR= 3.13 and 2.68 respectively) with an earlier introduction of solids compared to a high educational level (**Table 4**). Birth weight, birth order and gender were unrelated to the time of introducing solids in BF infants.

Discussion

In this sample some 37.2% of FF infants and 17.2 % of BF infants already received solids at the age of 4 completed months, although ESPGHAN and national recommendations in all participating countries advise not to introduce complementary foods before 4 months of age. Some 6.0% of FF infants, but only 0.6% of the BF infants, had introduced solids already at the age of 3 completed months. While introduction of solids is recommended at the same age for FF and BF infants, FF infants received solids much earlier than breastfed infants which is consistent with previous findings. (13;15;17). Our findings show that higher parental socioeconomic status and educational level, as well as exclusive breastfeeding during the first months of life, are associated with later introduction of complementary foods.

There are only few infants in whom solids are introduced later than recommended; 0.7% of FF infants and 2.3% of BF infants, respectively.

Our study involved 5 European countries with different cultural traditions and food patterns. Even though guidelines for the introduction of complementary foods are similar in these countries, there are significant differences in infant feeding practice between the countries, both in FF and BF infants (**Table 3 and 5**). We found much higher percentages of FF and BF infants with intake of solids at the age of 4 months in Belgium (**Table 3 and 5**). This earlier introduction, relative to other countries, is not due to different recommendations in Belgium and remains unexplained.

Giovannini et al. (19) studied infant feeding practices in Italy through the first year of life and found that 5.6% and 34.2% of the infants had introduced solids before the age of 3 and 4 months, respectively. Stated factors explaining an early introduction of solid foods were the infants' bodyweight at 1 month of age and maternal smoking during pregnancy. We found similar proportions for our Italian FF infants (2.4% and 30.5%, **Table 3**) although they had the lowest proportions of FF infants in our study with introduction of solids in the first 3 months of life.

German FF and BF infants had the lowest percentage in intake of solids at the age of 4 to 6 months. The proportion of infants at the age of 3 completed (FF infants 5% and BF infants 0.0%) and 6 completed months (91.2% FF infants and 69.5% BF infants) were lower compared to data from an earlier prospective study in German infants by Koletzko et al. (20) with 16% and 97% German infants consuming some Beikost (solid and liquid complementary food) at 3 and 6 months, respectively, while the German DONALD study reported 5% and 97% of the BF and 33% and 80% of the non BF infants to receive solids at the ages of 3 and 6 months, respectively. (21)

Other studies also reported discrepancies between feeding recommendations and practice. In the Euro-Growth Study, 50%, 67%, and 95% of infants were fed some solid foods at the ages of 3, 4, and 5 months, respectively. (22) In the United Kingdom the Department of Health recommendations suggests to start with complementary food between 4 to 6 months of age. Similarly, the Scientific Advisory Committee on Nutrition (SACN) commented that complementary food should not be introduced before the end of the fourth month (23). However, many infants receive complementary feeding earlier (13;22;24;25).

In this study, the strongest risk factors for early introduction of solids in FF infants at 3 completed months were country of residence and young maternal age, and at 4 months the country of residence, low maternal education and maternal smoking. In BF infants the country of residence and lower maternal education level were associated with introduction of solids at the age of 4 completed months. These findings are consistent with other studies also finding earlier introduction of complementary feeding in children of lower parental educational level

(26), lower socio economic status (14), maternal smoking (27) (16) and younger maternal age (12).

While we found no differences in the timing of introducing complementary foods between our infants from the intervention group fed formulae with different protein and fat contents, there were significant differences between countries in the timing of introducing complementary foods. This observation suggests far stronger effects of cultural, social and parental factors on the time of introducing complementary foods rather than of the dietary macronutrient composition.

More normal foods (NF) than commercial infant products (CIP) were given to breastfed infants during the first year of life, whereas a higher percentage of FF infants consumed CIP than NF. It seems that breastfeeding mothers prefer normal foods to commercial prepared or semi-prepared products; however, mothers of infants who feed formula and, hence, are already using a commercial product may tend to have a lower threshold for introducing other commercial products into the infants diet.

Conclusions

Infants given formula milk started solids significantly earlier than breastfed infants. There are marked differences between the 5 European countries of our study in the timing of introducing solids. The macronutrient composition of our formula milk groups did not influence the time point of introduction of complementary foods. Only few infants start complementary feeding later than recommended. Given the increasing evidence that early nutrition and growth has marked effects both on short-term but also long-term health, further studies should evaluate strategies to improve complementary feeding practice in populations of healthy infants.

Acknowledgements

We are extremely grateful to the parents and their infants who participated in this study, and to the physicians, midwifes and nurses for their helpful support in recruiting mothers during pregnancy or after giving birth. We want to thank the CHOP team for their effort and dedication, the dieticians for the patience to complete the nutritional data and Fabio Confalionieri for his support of the NutrCalc software. The European Childhood Obesity Programme is being carried out with financial support of the European Community, under the 5th Framework Programme for Research, Technology & Demonstration „Quality of Life and

Management of Living Resources", Key Action 1 (Food, Nutrition & Health), contract number QLK1-CT2002-389.

Funding

The study was supported in part by the Comission of the European Communities, specific RTD Programme "Quality of Life and Management of Living Resources", within the 5th Framework Programme (research grant no. QLRT-2001-00389 and QLK1-CT-2002-30582) and the 6th Framework Programme (contract no.007036); the Child Health Foundation, Munich, Germany; LMU innovative research priority project MC-Health (sub-project I); the Competence Network Obesity funded by the German Federal Ministry of Education and Research (FKZ 01GIo828); and the International Danone Institutes. Berthold Koletzko is the recipient of a Freedom to Discover Award of the Bristol Myers Squibb Foundation, New York, NY, USA. The presented data are part of the PhD Thesis in Human Biology submitted by Sonia Schiess to the medical faculty, Ludwig-Maximilians-University of Munich.

The authors report no conflicts of interest.

Reference List

1. WHO 54th World Health Assembly. Infant and young child nutrition. WHA54.2. 2001.
2. WHO. Complementary feeding of young children in developing countries: A review of current scientific knowledge. WHO 1998;WHO/NUT/98.1.
3. ESPGHAN Committee of Nutrition: Agostoni C, Decsi T, Fewtrell M et al. Complementary feeding: a commentary by the ESPGHAN Committee on Nutrition. J Pediatr Gastroenterol Nutr 2008;46:99-110.
4. Greer FR, Sicherer SH, Burks AW, and the Committee on Nutrition and Section on Allergy and Immunology. Effects of Early Nutritional Interventions on the Development of Atopic Disease in Infants and Children: The Role of Maternal Dietary Restriction, Breastfeeding, Timing of Introduction of Complementary Foods, and Hydrolyzed Formulas. Pediatrics 2008;121:183-91.
5. Kersting M. Ernährung des gesunden Säuglings. Monatsschrift Kinderheilkunde 2001;149:4-10.

6. Wirth S, Böhles H, Höger P, et al. Leitlinien Kinder- und Jugendmedizin der Deutschen Gesellschaft für Kinder- und Jugendmedizin. München, Urban&Fischer 2007.
7. O.N.E. The nouveaux aliments en douceur. Danièle Lecleir. 2000.
8. Società Italiana di Neonatologia. Raccomandazioni sull'allattamento materno per i nati a termine, di peso appropriato, sani. Medico e Bambino 2002;21:91-8.
9. Ksiazyk J, Rudzka-Kantoch Z, Weker H. Feeding plan for breast-fed infants and non-breast-fed infants. Medycyna Praktyczna Pediatria 2001;5:1-2.
10. Ksiazyk J, Rudzka-Kantoch Z, Weker H. Zalecenia zywienia niemowlat. Standardy Medyczne 2001;7/8:3:10-6.
11. Lázaro Almarza A, Marín-Lázaro JF. Alimentación del lactante sano. www aeped es/protocolos/nutricion/2 pdf 2001.
12. Savage SA, Reilly JJ, Edwards CA, Durnin JVGA. Weaning practice in the Glasgow longitudinal infant growth study. Arch Dis Child 1998;79:153-6.
13. Wright CM, Parkinson KN, Drewett RF. Why are babies weaned early? Data from a prospective population based cohort study. Arch Dis Child 2004;89:813-6.
14. Alder EM, Williams FL, Anderson AS, Forsyth S, Florey C, van der Velde P. What influence the timing of the introduction of solid food to infants ? British Journal of Nutrition 2004;92(3):527-31.
15. Lande.B., Andersen.L.F., Baerug A et al. Infant feeding practices and associated factors in the first six months of life: The Norwegian Infant Nutrition Survey. Acta Paediatr 2003;92:152-61.
16. Ford RP, Schluter PJ, Mitchell EA. Factors associated with the age of introduction of solids into the diet of new Zealand infants. New Zealand Cot Death Study Group. J Paediatr Child Health 1995;31(5):469-72.
17. van den Boom.S.A.M., Kimber AC, Morgan JB. Weaning practices in children up to 19 months of age in Madrid. Acta Paediatr 1995;84:853-8.
18. Koletzko B, von Kries R, Monasterolo RC et al. Lower protein in infant formula is associated with lower weight up to age 2 years: a randomized clinical trial. Am J Clin Nutr 2009;89:1-10.
19. Giovannini M, Riva E, Banderali G et al. Feeding practices of infants through the first year of life in Italy. Acta Paediatr 2004;93:492-7.

20. Koletzko B, Dokoupil K, Reitmayr S, Weimert-Harendza B, Keller E. Dietary fat intakes in infants and primary school children in Germany. Am J Clin Nutr 2000;72:1392S-1398.
21. Hilbig A, Kersting M. Effects of age and time on energy and macronutrient intake in German infants and young children: results of the DONALD Study. J Pediatr Gastroenterol Nutr 2006;43:518-24.
22. Freeman V, Van´t Hof M, Haschke F. Patterns of milk and food intake in infants from birth to age 36 months: the Euro-Growth Study. J Pediatr Gastroenterol Nutr 2000;31 Suppl 1:S76-S85.
23. Foote KD, Marriott LD. Weaning of infants. Arch Dis Child 2003;88:488-92.
24. Anderson AS, Guthrie CA, Alder EM, Forsyth S, Howie PW, Williams FLR. Rattling the plate--reasons and rationales for early weaning. Health Educ Res 2001;16:471-9.
25. Reilly JJ, Wells JCK. Duration of exclusive breast-feeding: introduction of complementary feeding may be necessary before 6 months of age. British Journal of Nutrition 2005;94:869-72.
26. Hendricks K, Briefel R, Novak T, Ziegler P. Maternal and Child Characteristics Associated with Infant and Toddler Feeding Practices. Journal of the American Dietetic Association 2006;106:135-48.
27. Ratner PA, Johnson JL, Bottorff JL. Smoking Relapse and Early Weaning Among Postpartum Women: Is There an Association? Birth 1999;26:76-82.

Table 1: Study participants and their socio-demographic characteristics

		N	Formula fed (FF) n	Formula fed (FF) %	Breast fed (BF) n	Breast fed (BF) %	p value
Total		1366	928	67.9	438	32.1	
Country	Germany	233	159	68.2	74	31.8	
	Belgium	180	108	60.0	72	40.0	
	Italy	370	220	59.5	150	40.5	
	Poland	222	169	76.1	53	23.9	
	Spain	361	272	75.3	89	24.7	$p<0.001$
Gender	male		475	70.1	203	29.9	
	female		453	65.8	235	34.2	n.s.
Both parents foreigner	yes		42	66.7	21	33.3	n.s.
Mother's education level	no/low		290	87.1	43	12.9	
	middle		482	70	207	30	
	high		153	44.9	188	55.1	$p<0.001$
Father's education level	no/low		305	81.6	69	18.4	
	middle		467	71.2	189	28.8	
	high		136	43.2	179	56.8	$p<0.001$
Smoking anytime	yes		417	81.6	94	18.4	$p<0.001$
Smoking during pregnancy	yes		386	83.9	74	16.1	$p<0.001$
Smoked up to the day pregnancy confirmed	yes		380	83.7	74	16.3	$p<0.001$
Smoked last 3 months prior pregnancy	yes		416	81.7	93	18.3	$p<0.001$
Smoked further (beyond 12th week)	yes		259	90.9	26	9.1	$p<0.001$
Birth order	1st child		511	65.6	268	34.4	
	2nd child		306	69.7	133	30.3	
	3rd child		82	71.3	33	28.7	
	>3rd child		26	89.7	3	10.3	$p<0.05$
Mother working at the end of month 1	yes		40	76.9	12	23.1	$p<0.05$

Figure 1: Cumulative percentage of formula fed and breast fed children with introduction of solids, per month

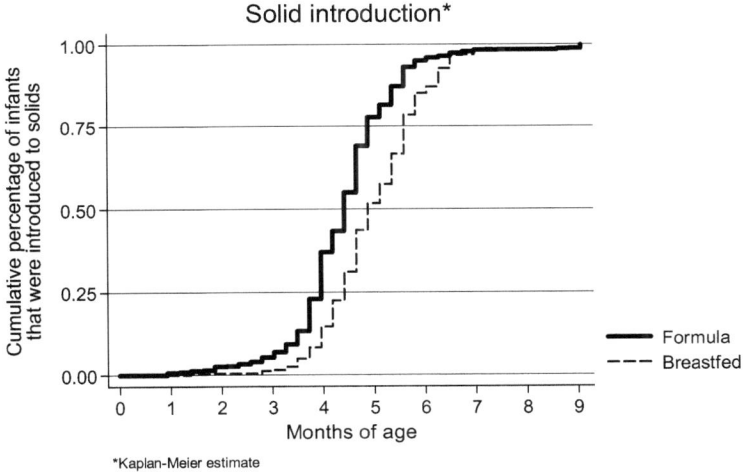

*Kaplan-Meier estimate

Table 2: Age, number and percentage of formula fed and breast fed infants with introduction of commercial infant products (CIP) and normal food (NF)

Age completed month	Total N	FF infants			BF infants		
		n	CIP (%)	NF (%)	n	CIP (%)	NF (%)
1	1045	696	27.6	22.8	349	5.4	7.7
2	1208	847	31.8	23.6	361	5.3	8.0
3	1184	847	32.0	26.1	337	6.5	8.3
4	1136	806	51.4	40.4	330	17.3	19.1
5	1128	796	77.1	63.6	332	45.2	49.4
6	1075	757	93.3	79.3	318	77.0	79.9
7	1008	705	97.0	89.6	303	93.4	93.7
8	984	695	97.4	91.9	289	95.8	97.6
9	967	682	97.2	95.5	285	97.2	98.6
12	945	658	96.7	99.2	287	93.0	100.0

Table 3: Numbers and cumulative percentage of formula fed infants receiving solids, by age and country

Age month completed	Germany n	%	Belgium n	%	Italy n	%	Poland n	%	Spain n	%
1**	1	0.0	5	5.3	0	0.0	2	3.1	2	0.9
2***	6	4.3	10	9.9	1	0.5	4	2.5	4	1.7
3***	7	5.0	15	15.8	5	2.4	5	3.1	19	7.8
4**	41	31.3	50	55.6	61	30.5	60	39.0	88	38.1
5***	85	67.5	66	75.0	162	81.4	145	94.2	184	80.3
6**	114	91.2	75	93.8	190	98.4	142	97.3	207	97.2
7**	115	96.6	69	100.0	190	100.0	127	100.0	199	99.5
8**	107	96.4	71	100.0	187	99.5	127	100.0	198	100.0
9	109	100.0	74	100.0	182	99.5	129	100.0	187	100.0
12	101	100.0	67	100.0	180	100.0	132	100.0	178	100.0

* $<p\ 0.05$, ** $p<0.01$, *** $p<0.001$

Table 4. Variables significantly associated with the timing of introduction of solids to formula fed and breast fed infants, at age of 3 and 4 months[†]

			FF infants multiple logistic regression		BF infants multiple logistic regression			
Age 3 months	n	%	OR	95% CI	N	%	OR	95% CI
Germany[‡]	7	5	1.00		0	0.0	1.00	
Belgium	15	15.6	3.96	1.47-10.67 *	0	0.0		
Italy	5	2.4			1	0.6		
Poland	5	3.1			0	0.0		
Spain	19	7.8			1	1.4		
Mother's age								
≤ 25 years	17	11.3	2.86	1.01-8.05 *	0	0.0	1.00	
>25-30 years	14	5.1			2	6.7		
>30-35 years	14	6.1			0	0.0		
>35 years[‡]	6	4.1	1.00		2	1.4		
Mother's education level								
no/low	19	7.4			0	0.0	1.00	
middle	25	5.7			2	6.7		
high[‡]	6	4.1	1.00		0	0.0		
Smoking mother								
yes	28	7.6			0	0.0		
no[‡]	23	4.9	1.00		2	0.8	1.00	
Age 4 months								
Germany[‡]	41	31.3	1.00		3	4.9	1.00	
Belgium	50	55.6	3.28	1.83-5.86 ***	16	43.2	15.93	3.99-63.62 ***
Italy	61	30.5			17	14.7		
Poland	60	39.0			3	8.7		
Spain	88	38.1			18	25.7	6.60	1.80-24.20 *
Mother's age								
≤ 25 years	62	45.3			7	26.9		
>25-30 years	113	43.1			16	18.2		
>30-35 years	87	32.7			23	16.5		
>35 years[‡]	38	27.1	1.00		11	14.5	1.00	
Mother's education level								
no/low	108	43.8	1.87	1.47-3.08 *	9	26.1	3.16	1.08-9.04 *
middle	150	35.5			33	21.4	2.66	1.24-5.79 *
high[‡]	43	30.7	1.00		15	10.5	1.00	
Smoking mother								
yes	143	42.6	1.40	1.04-1.92 *	17	24.5		
no[‡]	150	33.2	1.00		40	15.4	1.00	

[†] Variables assessed to be included in the model were country of residence, mother's age, mother's educational level, and maternal smoking habit. [‡] Reference group * p<0.05, *** p<0.005

Table 5: Numbers and cumulative percentage of breast fed infants receiving solids, by age and country

Age month completed	Germany n	%	Belgium n	%	Italy n	%	Poland n	%	Spain n	%
1	0	0.0	0	0.0	0	0.0	0	0.0	2	2.5
2	1	1.4	0	0.0	1	0.7	0	0.0	0	0.0
3	0	0.0	0	0.0	1	0.8	0	0.0	1	1.4
4***	3	4.9	16	43.2	17	14.7	3	6.7	18	25.7
5***	15	25.0	39	84.8	65	58.6	17	36.2	47	70.1
6***	41	69.5	46	95.8	102	92.7	37	84.1	51	89.5
7	54	93.1	48	100.0	102	99.0	39	97.5	53	98.1
8	57	100.0	41	100.0	98	97.0	42	100.0	47	97.9
9	55	100.0	44	100.0	98	99.0	41	100.0	46	100.0
12	50	100.0	46	100.0	101	100.0	41	100.0	48	100.0

* $p<0.05$, ** $p<0.01$, *** $p<0.001$

Intake of energy providing liquids during the first year of life in five European countries

Sonia A Schiess[1], Veit Grote[2], Silvia Scaglioni[3], Veronica Luque[4], Francoise Martin[5], Anna Stolarczyk[6], Fiammetta Vecchi[3], Berthold Koletzko[1],
for the European Childhood Obesity Project *

[1]Div. Metabolic and Nutritional Medicine, Dr. von Hauner Children's Hospital, University of Munich Medical Centre, München, Germany, [2] Dept. Epidemiology, Inst. of Social Paediatrics and Adolescent Medicine, University of Munich, München, Germany [3]Dept. of Paediatrics, San Paolo Hospital, University of Milan, Italy, [4]Paediatrics Research Unit, University Rovira i Virgili, Reus, Spain, [5]CHC St. Vincent, Rocourt, Belgium, [6]Clinic of Paediatrics, Children's Memorial Health Institute, Warsaw, Poland

*Study team: **Belgium** (ULB Bruxelles and CHC St Vincent Liège): Carlier C, Goyens P, Hoyos J, Langhendries J-P, Martin F, Van Hees J-N, Xhonneux A; **Germany** (Division of Paediatric Epidemiology, Institute of Social Pediatrics and Adolescent Medicine and Division of Nutritional Medicine and Metabolism, Dr. von Hauner Children's Hospital, Ludwig Maximilians University of Munich): Beyer J, Demmelmair H, Fritsch M, Handel U, Hannibal I, Kreichauf S, von Kries R, Pawellek I, Verwied-Jorky S; **Italy** (University of Milan): Giovannini M, Agostoni C, Confalonieri F, Scaglioni S, Tedeschi S, Vecchi F, Verduci E; **Spain** (Universitat Rovira i Virgili): Closa Monasterolo R, Escribano Subias J, Méndez Riera G, Luque Moreno V; **Poland** (Children's Memorial Health Institute): Socha J, Dobrzańska A, Gruszfeld D, Socha P, Stolarczyk A, Janas R, Pietraszek E, Kowalik A

Published in Clinical Nutrition 29 (2010); 726-732

List of abbreviations

AAP	American Academy of Paediatrics
EPL	Energy providing liquids
BF	breast fed
FF	formula fed
ESPGHAN	European Society for Paediatric Gastroenterology, Hepatology and Nutrition

Abstract

Background: Intake of energy providing liquids (EPL) other than breast milk or formula to infants is discouraged because it may displace milk intake. Data on actual practice is lacking.

Aim: To describe the current practice of EPL supply to infants in five European countries.

Method: Breastfed (BF) infants and infants fed using two formulas (FF) with different protein content were recruited from October 2002 to June 2004. Three-day weighed food protocols of 1368 infants were obtained monthly at the ages of 1 to 9 and again at 12 completed months.

Results: At the age of 4 months, 13% of BF and 43% of FF infants received EPL. FF infants started EPL earlier (median 17 weeks) than BF infants (median 30 weeks). EPL intake was associated with a lower intake of formula milk and solids (kcal/d) in the first year of life. Multiple regression analysis showed significant differences in EPL introduction between the individual countries.

Conclusion: In contrast to recommendations, EPL is frequently given during the first months of life to breastfed and particularly to formula fed infants. Infants given EPL showed lower intakes of infant formula and solids. Caregivers should receive better counselling on appropriate infant feeding.

Introduction

Healthy infants should preferably be breastfed and should not receive complementary foods (solids and liquids other than breast milk, infant formula or follow-on formula) in addition to breastfeeding (or formula feeding) before 17 weeks nor later than 26 weeks of age[1];[2]. Infants do not require additional liquids like water, tea, juices, sweetened beverages or other energy providing liquids (EPL) other than breast milk or infant formula during at least the first half year of life, with the possible exception of selected conditions such as diarrhoea, very high ambient temperatures, high fever or other excessive fluid losses, or in some selected indications occurring in the neonatal period [3].

The provision of EPL during the first year of life is not recommended. Feeding infants with EPL may displace breast milk or infant formula intake and, thereby, may adversely affect nutrient supply[4]. Moreover, infants with regular intake of EPL might be primed to their sweet taste with a possible increased risk for later development of dental caries or obesity [4];[5];[6];[7]. High intakes of fruit juice can exceed the capacity for fructose absorption and induce diarrhoea, abdominal pain and growth faltering[8];[9];[10];[4].

The American Academy of Paediatrics (AAP) concluded that fruit juices have no nutritional advantages over whole fruit; they lack fibre, are consumed more quickly and do not promote the desirable behaviour of eating whole fruits[4]. The AAP recommended to provide fruit juices only after the age of 6 months when infants can drink from a cup, and only as part of a meal in order to reduce the risk of dental caries induction[4], whereas others recommended not providing fruit juice before the age of 9 months[11]. In contrast to these recommendations, an increasing use of fruit juices in the infant diet has been reported[12]. Sales of juices for infants in the United States increased from 9.7% of total complementary feeding products in 1971 to 16.7% in 1984 and probably further by 1992[12].

There is a lack of current data on EPL consumption by infants. We aimed to characterize the practice of introducing EPL to infants in five European countries with similar infant feeding recommendations. Data was collected as part of the prospective European Childhood Obesity Project. We explored whether type of milk feeding, socio-demographic characteristics and the country of residence were associated with EPL use, and whether EPL consumption influences the intake of infant formula or solids.

Subjects and Methods
Study design
Data were collected as part of the European Childhood Obesity Project, a double-blind, randomized controlled trial with one group of breastfed (BF) infants and two groups of formula fed (FF) infants randomized to formula with different protein levels as a possible risk factor for later obesity. The methodology of the study has been previously reported[13];[14]. In short, eligible participants were healthy, singletons, term infants recruited between 1 October 2002 to 31 June 2004 and followed-up in 11 study centres in 5 European countries (Belgium, Germany, Italy, Poland and Spain). Mothers were contacted at maternity hospitals by trained study personnel, or after hospital discharge by midwives or paediatricians.

After receiving oral and written information of the study and providing written consent, parents were invited to the first medical visit for collection of socioeconomic data, medical history of parents and infant, and infant anthropometry. During the following months, parents and infants were followed at regular intervals in the study centres, as well as by mailed questionnaires on feeding behaviours.

Dietary intervention
A reference group of infants fully breastfed for at least 3 months (BF) was followed without any intervention. Formula fed infants (FF) were randomized not later than 8 weeks of age to receive two infant formulae and later follow-on formulae with either higher or lower protein levels for the duration of the first year of life[14]. There was no other intervention with respect to the infant diet.

Data collection
All data other than food protocols were collected by standardized questionnaires. A 3-day weighed food protocol was chosen to collect detailed information on the infant food and nutrient intake. Parents were asked to complete weighed food protocol on 3 consecutive days, including 2 week days and one weekend day, monthly at the ages of 1 to 9 completed months and again at 12 months. Volumes of milk were recorded based on the scale in the feeding bottles. Other food items were weighed on a digital food scale with an accuracy of 1 g (Soehnle unica, No. 66006, Nassau, Germany) given to the parents at the 3-month study visit. Parents were asked to record the time and place of feeding, the intake of all milk, liquid and solid food; for FF infants, the quantity (grams) of water, milk powder or cereals used for the preparation of each formula bottle, the amount (ml) of formula milk offered and the amount actually consumed by the infant. Parents were requested to note

any intake of liquid other than breast or infant formula, the product and brand name of the liquid, and the time when it was first introduced. All other food items, their brand names or the recipe in case of home prepared foods, the quantity (grams) of food offered and the quantity consumed by the infant, were recorded. Trained dieticians in all study centres entered the data of the food protocols from their centre using a special software developed for this study. Nutrient content data of foods was derived from the German Food Code and Nutrient data base Bundeslebensmittelschlüssel, BLS II.3 (Federal Institute for Risk Assessment, Berlin, Germany). Nutrient contents of new food items as well as country specific foods were added to the data base as required. Standard Operating Procedures (SOPS) were developed and implemented, and dietary study staff participated in semi-annual training workshops to ensure consistent procedures and quality for data introduction and calculations in all participating centres.

We were unable to measure breast milk volume intake in the study population of the 5 countries under the conditions of the study.

The two infant formula groups with different protein levels did not differ in the intake of EPL, fruit juice, vegetable juice or instant tea. Therefore, we choose to describe the results on EPL intake for the combined group of all formula fed infants.

Definition of energy providing liquids (EPL)

Complementary foods (3281 food items) consumed during the first year of life by the infants in the 5 countries were classified by their ingredients and categorized into subgroups. For this analysis, EPL were defined as sugared instant tea, fruit juices (100% fruit juice, fruit drinks), vegetable juices provided as drinks (but not as one ingredient of a composed dish), and other sugared beverages (soft drinks, sugared water without or with flavours).

Socio-demographic data

Mothers were categorized into three education levels (low= preliminary to lower secondary, middle=upper secondary and post-secondary, and high=first and second stage of tertiary education) and by age at birth (I= ≤25, II= >25 to 30, III= > 30 to 35 and IV= > 35 years).

Statistics

All analyses were stratified by feeding type (breastfed / formula fed). Chi-square test and multiple logistic regression were used to analyse the time points of EPL introduction. We applied multiple logistic regression models for each month to detect associations between maternal age, education level, smoking behaviour, country of residence and times of introducing EPL. Wilcoxon rank-sum tests were performed to compare the energy intakes of infants with and without EPL consumption. Stata 9.2, SPSS 16.0 and Excel 2000 were used for data analysis.

Ethics

The study protocol was reviewed and accepted by the ethic committees at all study centres.

Results

At least one informative 3-day weighed food protocol was available for 1368 infants (82% of the 1678 infants recruited). Of the 1184 children with food protocols still participating in the study at 6 months, 875 (74%) completed all 6 monthly food protocols until this age.

BF infants

Some 75% of BF infants received EPL during the first year of life. The median age at introduction was 30 weeks. Ten percent of breastfed infants received EPL at 9 weeks, 8% to 10% of the BF infants received **EPL** (mostly instant tea) during the first 3 months of life (**Figure 1A**). From 4 to 6 completed months, the proportion of BF infants introduced to EPL increased from 13% to 36%.

There were marked differences in EPL consumption between countries (**Figure 2A**). At the age of 1 month, 8% of BF infants in Italy, 14% in Poland and 10% in Spain, received EPL. At 3 months we found the highest proportions of infants with EPL intake in Poland and Italy and at 4 to 9 months in Poland and Spain.

Also the type of EPL consumed differed considerably between the countries. Not more than 10% of the BF infants in Germany, Belgium and Spain consumed **instant tea** during the first year of life, whereas 56 % of BF infants in Poland and 29% in Italy received instant tea (**Table S1**).

At the age of 4 completed months 7% of BF infants received **fruit juice.** Early introduction (mainly orange juice) was seen especially in Spain, where 23% of all infants received some at the age of 4 completed months (**Table S1**). The highest proportions of BF infants with an intake of fruit juice were found in the second half of the year in Poland (34% to 66%) and Spain (44% to 61%), and at the end of the first year in Germany (58%), whereas Italian infants showed the lowest proportion (13% to 29%) (data not shown). **Vegetable juice** (mostly carrot juice) was consumed almost exclusively by Polish and German BF infants (**Table S1**). No BF infants had received vegetable juice until the age of 4 months while 2% of

BF infants in Belgium, 7% in Germany and 16% in Poland consumed some vegetable juice at the age of 6 months.

Beverages like soft drinks or sugar-added flavoured waters were hardly consumed at all by BF infants (<0.5 %) during the first year of life.

Applying a multiple logistic regression for each month on the introduction of EPL in BF infants during the first 7 months of life, including the effects of maternal age, education level, smoking behaviour and country of residence, the main predicting factor for introduction of EPL was consistently the country of residence (**Table 1**). Polish BF infants had a 17-fold higher odds to consume EPL at the age of 3 months than BF infants in Germany. Also, in Italy, we found a 10-fold higher risk for BF infants to receive EPL at the age of 3 months, and in Spain at the age of 4 months, as compared to BF infants in Germany.

We repeated the same analytical approach for instant tea, fruit and vegetable juice. In addition to the effect of country of residence, a low maternal educational level was associated with introduction of EPL and instant tea at the age of 3 completed months (OR 4.3, CI: 1.3-14.0, p=0.17), and maternal smoking was associated with introduction of fruit juice at 4 (OR 3.2, CI: 1.0-9.8, p=0.04) and 6 completed months (OR 2.2, CI: 1.1-4.3, p=0.02) (data not shown).

FF infants

During the first year of life, 86% of FF infants received **EPL** and the median age at introduction was 17 weeks. Some 30.0% of FF infants received EPL at the age of one month and 43% and 57% at the ages of 4 and 6 completed months, respectively. During the first 4 months, instant tea, with up to 33% of the infants, was the predominant EPL consumed by the FF infants (**Figure 1B**). Fruit juices (mainly apple and orange juice) were given to 31% of FF infants at 5 months and up to 46% during the following months. Some 5% of all the FF infants consumed vegetable juice (mainly carrot juice or mixtures of carrot juice with fruit juice) at 4 months, and less than 10% during the rest of the year. Other sugared beverages were hardly consumed by FF infants at all (<0.5%).

We found significant differences between the countries in EPL consumption (**Figure 2B**). During the first 4 months of life, infants in Poland had the highest proportion receiving EPL (79% to 88%), followed by Germany (35% to 44%), Italy (25% to 33%), Spain (22% to 35%) and Belgium (1% to 12%).

Instant teas were consumed by 88% of FF infants in Poland at the age of one month, and between 70% and 88% during the first year of life (**Table S2**). During the first 4 months of life,

28% to 32% of FF infants in Germany, 25% to 31% in Italy and 26% to 13% in Spain consumed some instant tea. In Spain, this proportion declined over the year and, in Belgium, less than 5% of all FF infants received instant tea.

At the age of 4 months 14% of FF infants consumed some **fruit juice**. Italy (0% to 29%) had the lowest proportion of infants getting fruit juice during the first year, whereas infants in Germany (2% to 3%) and Spain (2% to 8%) already received fruit juice during the first 3 months of life (**Table S2**). At the age of 4 months (17 weeks), 10% FF infants in Germany, 11% in Belgium, 20% in Poland and 24% in Spain consumed some fruit juice. In Italy, only 2% of the FF infants consumed fruit juice at 4 months and 10% at 6 months, as compared to 39% - 54% in the other countries. **Vegetable juice** was consumed by Polish and German FF infants between the ages of 3 and 12 completed months, but hardly in other countries (**Table S2**). Applying a multiple logistic regression model for each of the first 7 months, including maternal age, education level, smoking behaviour and country of residence as covariates for the introduction of EPL or instant tea in FF infants during the first year of life, country of residence was the only consistent predictive factor for an earlier introduction of EPL (in all months, p<0.001, **Table 1**). Compared to Germany, FF infants in Poland had an approximately 6 to 14-fold higher risk for EPL intake. Repeating the analysis only with the introduction of fruit juice in FF infants, the country of residence was also seen to be a risk factor at the ages of 3 to 12 months (p<0.05). Intakes of any EPL were not associated with protein contents of study formula, birth weight or birth order. The two formula groups also did not differ regarding the consumption of fruit juice, vegetable juice or instant tea, with the only exception being a significantly higher fruit juice intake in the high protein group at the age of 5 months (p=0.026).

Applying a multiple regression for the first 4 months of life including the effect of country of residence, maternal age and educational level as well as the maternal smoking behaviour, we found that FF infants were 5 times more likely to receive EPL up to 4 months of age (OR:5.1; 95%CI: 4.1-6.3).

Energy providing liquid and energy intake

Table 2 shows the total energy intake (kcal/d), the energy intake from EPL, formula milk and solids of FF infants with and without EPL consumption. FF infants receiving EPL had a significantly lower energy supply through infant formula at the ages of 2 to 5 months. This is also seen in **Table S3** where the median intake of EPL (ml/d), as well as the intake of infant formula (ml/d) in FF infants with and without EPL, are shown. At the ages of 4 and 5 months, infants receiving EPL consumed a significantly higher energy intake from solids than infants without EPL consumption. But infants with EPL consumption had a significantly lower energy intake from solids at the ages of 7 to 9 and at 12 completed months.

Discussion

This study shows that EPL are given to a very high proportion of European infants during the first months of life. Some 13% of BF infants and 43% of FF infants receive EPL by the age of 4 months, even though such a practice is not supported at all by current recommendations[2]. There is no nutritional benefit of feeding EPL or fruit juices to infants during the first months of life, but there is a possible risk of displacing nutrient intakes from breast milk or infant formula[15],[16],[17]. Our data analysis revealed a lower formula milk intake (kcal/d) in FF infants who consumed EPL during the first months of life. Furthermore, infants who consumed EPL had a lower solids intake (kcal/d) during the second half of the first year. The significantly lower infant formula intake in infants with EPL coincides with the time of the highest percentage of infants with instant tea intake as EPL. This is of concern, since instant tea provides only rapidly absorbable carbohydrates and none of the essential nutrients supplied with breast milk or infant formula.

Infants who received EPL had significantly higher energy intakes from solids at the ages of 4 and 5 months as compared to infants who did not receive EPL, suggesting that the provision of EPL is associated with an earlier solid introduction in the infant's diet.

There are markedly different feeding practices between the countries. Both in FF and BF infants, country of residence is a consistent predictive factor for the time of EPL introduction (**Table 1**). These country differences might be due to differences in local traditions of infant feeding or in communication to parents, but are not explained by infant feeding recommendations which are similar throughout these five countries.

Our findings also show that FF infants receive EPL and solids earlier and to a higher proportion then BF infants, although the recommendations do not differ[18],[19]. Up to the age of 4 months, FF infants were 5 times more likely to receive EPL than BF infants. Parada et al. also found higher consumption frequencies of tea and juices among bottle fed than among breastfed infants in Brazil during the first months of life[20]. Similarly, Emmett et al. found a higher percentage of British FF infants than BF infants receiving additional drinks other than breast milk or infant formula, and they speculated that this could be due to FF infants being accustomed to drinking from bottles[21].

In our study group, instant teas were the predominate form of EPL during the first months of life, whereas fruit and vegetable juices were increasingly introduced from 3 to 4 completed months onwards and consumed in higher proportions during the second half of the first year (**Figure 1+2**). Instant teas might be used in young infants with excessive crying, based on the assumption that infants should get some liquid in addition to breast milk or formula, whereas older infants might get fruit juice as a nutritional supplement or because it may be perceived to be more similar to complementary foods given at older ages. Parada et al. found higher percentages of Brazilian infants with an intake of teas from birth to the age of 4 months (29% for BF infants and 47% for FF infants) compared to our infants, and even up to 69% of the infants with an intake of fruit juices during the second half of the first year[20]. In the Feeding Infants and Toddlers Study (FITS), Menella et al. analysed the foods fed to Hispanic and non-Hispanic infants in the United States, and found similar percentages of infants with fruit juice intake as we found for our FF infants, but a much higher proportion of infants who consumed vegetable juice, even compared to our highest percentage of infants with an intake of vegetable juice who were found in Poland[22].

Sweet drinks are not recommended in the infant diet because they contribute few nutrients other than energy, whereas appropriate intake of breast milk or infant formula as well as complementary foods should provide the infants with an adequate nutrient intake[2],[23],[24],[25],[26]. Educational level of the caregiver, affordability of products, consumption habits of parents, guidance by health care professionals, as well as product advertising and marketing all may influence the consumption habits of sweet drinks[27],[28],[15],[16].

In conclusion, this study shows that, in contrast to current recommendations, EPL are provided surprisingly early and at a surprisingly high rate to infants during the first year of life, particularly in FF infants. The provision of EPL is associated with a lower energy intake from infant formula, earlier introduction of solids, and less energy intake from solids during the second half of the first year of life. Infant feeding practices should be improved by informing health care professionals, parents, and manufacturers of infant food products.

Acknowledgements

We thank the families who participated in this study, and the collaborating physicians, midwives and nurses for their help in informing and recruiting families. We are very grateful to the study partners for their efforts, endurance and dedication to this work. The European Childhood Obesity Project is carried out with financial support of the European Community, under the 5th Framework Programme for Research, Technology & Demonstration "Quality of Life and Management of Living Resources", Key Action 1 (Food, Nutrition & Health), contract number QLK1-CT2002-389 and 6th Framework priority 5.4.3.1 Food quality and safety (Early nutrition programming - long-term follow up of efficacy and safety trials and integrated epidemiological, genetic, animal, consumer and economic research, EARNEST, Food-CT-2005-007036). It does not necessarily reflect the views of the Commission and in no way anticipates its future policy in this area. Berthold Koletzko is the recipient of a Freedom to Discover Award of the Bristol Myers Squibb Foundation, New York, NY, USA. The presented data are part of the PhD Thesis in Human Biology submitted by Sonia Schiess to the Medical Faculty, Ludwig-Maximilians-University of Munich.

Statement of authorship:

SSch was involved in enrolment of subjects, acquisition and introduction of data, data analysis and interpretation, manuscript writing. VG data management and data analysis, contributed to manuscript writing. SSc participated in study design and in conducting the study, contributed to manuscript writing. VL, FM, AS, FV were involved in enrolment of subjects, in conducting the study, acquisition and introduction of data, and contributed to manuscript writing. BK, principal investigator of the study, contributed to manuscript writing. All authors read and approved the final version of the article.

Notifications of Conflicts of Interest and Ethical Adherence

None of the authors has declared a conflict of interest. The project was reviewed and accepted by the Ethics Committee of the Bavarian Board of physicians.

Reference List

1. ESPGHAN Committee on Nutrition: Agostoni C, Braegger C et al. Breast-feeding: A Commentary by the ESPGHAN Committee on Nutrition. J Pediatr Gastroenterol Nutr 2009;49:112-25.

2. ESPGHAN Committee of Nutrition: Agostoni C, Decsi T, Fewtrell M et al. Complementary feeding: a commentary by the ESPGHAN Committee on Nutrition. J Pediatr Gastroenterol Nutr 2008;46:99-110.
3. Kersting M. Ernährung des gesunden Säuglings. Monatsschrift Kinderheilkunde 2001;149:4-10.
4. Committee on Nutrition. The Use and Misuse of Fruit Juice in Pediatrics. Pediatrics 2001;107:1210-3.
5. Ludwig DS, Peterson KE, Gortmaker SL. Relation between consumption of sugar-sweetened drinks and childhood obesity: a prospective, observational analysis. The Lancet 2001;357:505-8.
6. Malik VS, Schulze MB, Hu FB. Intake of sugar-sweetened beverages and weight gain: a systematic review. Am J Clin Nutr 2006;84:274-88.
7. Vartanian LR, Schwartz MB, Brownell KD. Effects of soft drink consumption on nutrition and health: a systematic review and meta-analysis. Am J Public Health 2007;97(4):667-75.
8. Lifschitz CH. Carbohydrate Absorption From Fruit Juices in Infants. Pediatrics 2000;105:e4.
9. Cole CR, Rising R, Lifshitz F. Consequences of Incomplete Carbohydrate Absorption From Fruit Juice Consumption in Infants. Arch Pediatr Adolesc Med 1999;153:1098-102.
10. Smith MM, Davis M, Chasalow FI, Lifshitz F. Carbohydrate Absorption From Fruit Juice in Young Children. Pediatrics 1995;95:340-4.
11. van der Merwe J, Kluyts M, Bowley N, Marais D. Optimizing the introduction of complementary foods in the infant's diet: a unique challenge in developing countries. Maternal and Child Nutrition 2007;3:259-70.
12. Fomon SJ. Infant Feeding in the 20th Century: Formula and Beikost. J Nutr 2001;131:409S-420.
13. Koletzko B, von Kries R, Monasterolo RC et al. Can infant feeding choices modulate later obesity risk? Am J Clin Nutr 2009;89(5):S1502-S1508.
14. Koletzko B, von Kries R, Monasterolo RC et al. Lower protein in infant formula is associated with lower weight up to age 2 y: a randomized clinical trial. Am J Clin Nutr 2009;89:1-10.
15. Marshall TLS, Broffitt B, Eichenberger-Gilmore J, Stumbo J. Beverage consumption and infant nutrition - Benefits of milk vs. juice. Nutrition Research Newsletter 2003.

16. Saalfield S, Jackson-Allen P. Biopsychosocial consequences of sweetened drink consumption in children 0-6 years of age. Pediatric Nursing 2006;32(5):460-71.
17. Gibson SA. Non-milk extrinsic sugars in the diets of pre-school children: association with intakes of micronutrients, energy, fat and NSP. British Journal of Nutrition 1997;78:367-78.
18. Fewtrell MS, Morgan JB, Duggan C et al. Optimal duration of exclusive breastfeeding: what is the evidence to support current recommendations? Am J Clin Nutr 2007;85:635S-638.
19. Schiess, S., Grote, V., Scaglioni, S, Luque, V., Martin, F., Stolarczyk, A, Vechi, F., and Koletzko, B. Introduction of complementary feeding in five European countries. J Pediatr Gastroenterol Nutr 49, 1-8.
20. Parada C, Carvalhaes MABL.Jamas MT. Complementary feeding practices to children during their first year of life. Rev Latino-am Enfermagem 2007;15(2):282-9.
21. Emmett, P., North, K., Noble, S., and ALSPAC Study Team. Types of drinks consumed by infants at 4 and 8 months of age: a descriptive study. Public Health Nutrition 3(2), 211-217.
22. Mennella J, Ziegler P, Briefel R, Novak T. Feeding Infants and Toddlers Study: The types of foods fed to Hispanic infants and toddlers. J Am Diet Assoc 2006;106:S96-S106.
23. Daelmans B, Martines J, Saadeh R. Conclusions of the global consultation on complementary feeding. Food and Nutrition Bulletin 2003;24(1):126-9.
24. Dewey, K. G., Lutter, Chessa, Martines, J., Daelmans, B., and WHO Global Consultation on Complementary Feeding. Guiding principles for complementary feeding of the breastfed child. 1-37.
25. Monte CMG, Giugliani ERJ. Recommendations for the complementary feeding of the breastfed child. J Pediatr (Rio J) 2004;80 (5Suppl):S131-S141.
26. WHO. Complementary feeding. 1-24.
27. FISHER JO, Mitchell DC, Smiciklas-Wright H, BIRCH LL. Maternal Milk Consumption Predicts the Tradeoff between Milk and Soft Drinks in Young Girls' Diets. J Nutr 2001;131:246-50.
28. Hendricks K, Briefel R, Novak T, Ziegler P. Maternal and Child Characteristics Associated with Infant and Toddler Feeding Practices. Journal of the American Dietetic Association 2006;106:135-48.

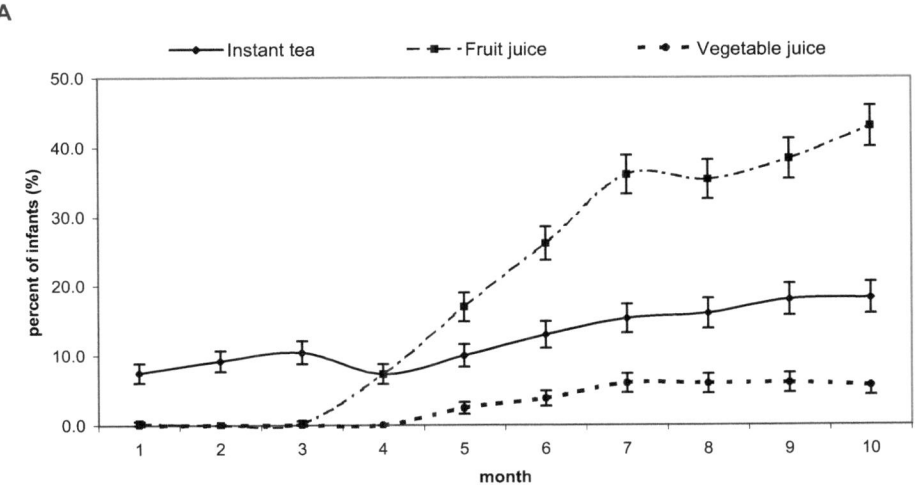

Figure 1: Percentage (%) and standard error (SE) of breastfed (**A**) and formula fed infants (**B**) with intake of instant tea, fruit juice or vegetable juice during the first year of life.

Figure 2. Percentage (%) and standard error (SE) of breastfed (A) and formula fed infants (B) with intake of energy providing liquid (EPL) by country, at the age of 1 to 9 and 12 completed months.

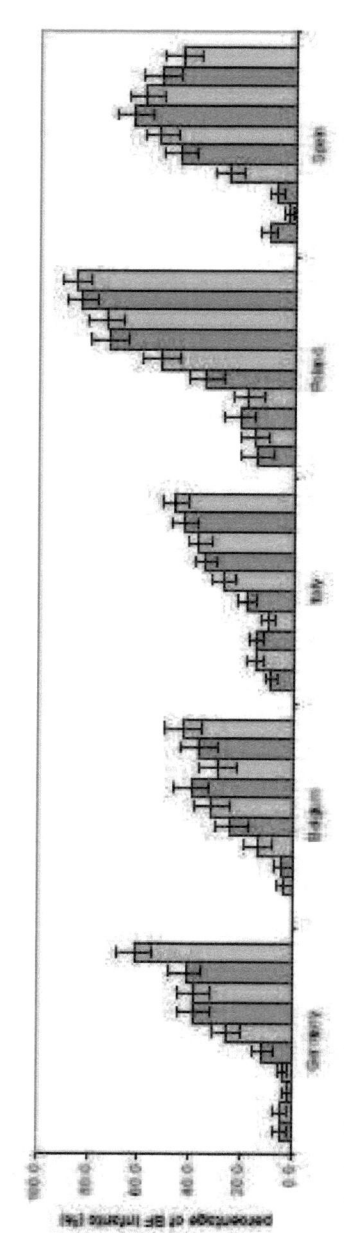

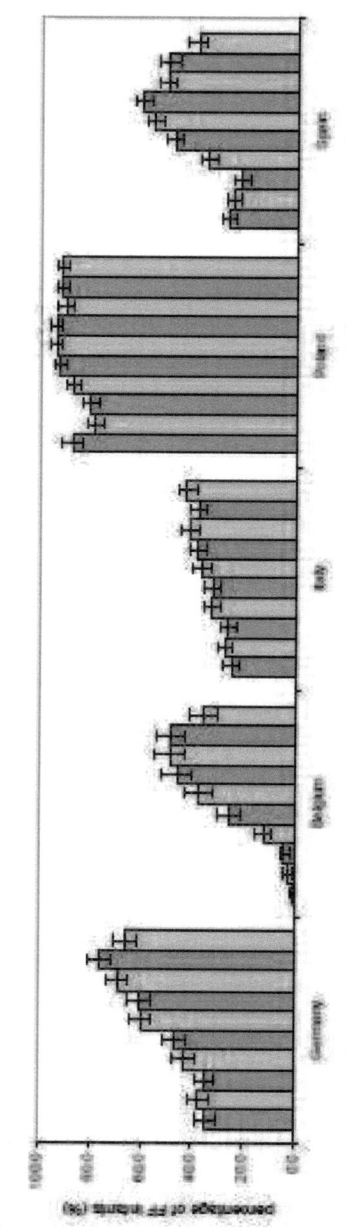

The proportion of breastfed infants with consumption of EPL differed significantly between the countries at the age of 2 to 12 completed months (all p<0.01).

The proportion of formula fed infants with consumption of EPL differed significantly between the countries at the age of 1 to 12 completed months (in all months p<0.05).

Table 1: Odds ratios (95% confidence interval) for the introduction of energy providing liquid in the countries compared to Germany (reference). Based on logistic regression for each age group (age of 1 to 7 completed months) including maternal age, maternal education level and maternal smoking behaviour.

Age (completed months)	Belgium			Italy			Poland			Spain		
	OR	95% CI	p-value	OR	95% CI	p-value	OR	95% CI	p-value	OR	95% CI	p-value
Breastfed infants												
1												
2				3.92	(1.08-14.17)	0.04						
3				9.94	(1.26-78.51)	0.03	17.71	(2.06-152.62)	0.01			
4							8.2	(1.57-42.85)	0.01	10.2	(2.23-46.70)	0.003
5							3.46	(1.14-9.84)	0.02	6.38	(2.49-16.38)	<0.001
6							3.4	(1.40-8.28)	0.01	3.13	(1.41-6.95)	0.01
7							3.53	(1.40-8.85)	0.01	2.74	(1.25-5.99)	0.01

Formula fed infants

1	0.02	(0.01-0.15)	<0.001	11.77	(5.03-27.54)	<0.001
2	0.05	(0.16-0.18)	<0.001	5.71	(3.36-9.70)	<0.001
3	0.09	(0.03-0.25)	<0.001	7.31	(4.22-12.68)	<0.001
4	0.2	(0.10-0.41)	<0.001	9.3	(4.54-15.17)	<0.001
5	0.44	(0.24-0.80)	0.01	14.13	(6.85-29.18)	<0.001
6	0.4	(0.22-0.72)	0.01	9.24	(4.24-20.12)	<0.001
7	0.43	(0.26-0.69)	<0.001	9.06	(3.97-20.66)	<0.001

0.53 (0.33-0.85) 0.01

Table 2: Intake of total energy (kcal/d), energy providing liquids (kcal/d), solids (kcal/d) and formula milk (kcal/d) by infants with and without intake of energy providing liquid (EPL), presented as median and interquartile range (IQR).

Age (completed months)	Infants with EPL intake			Infants without EPL intake			p value [a]
	N	Total energy intake (kcal/d) (median)	(IQR)	N	Total energy intake (kcal/d) (median)	(IQR)	
1	181	530	(450;586)	506	514	(445;575)	
2	275	560	(487;619)	633	548	(489;619)	
3	277	570	(508;637)	642	576	(522;643)	
4	330	618	(545;682)	570	611	(554;674)	
5	384	664	(602;740)	498	656	(581;712)	*
6	430	700	(612;794)	446	678	(610;762)	
7	394	743	(656;832)	417	747	(645;833)	
8	371	781	(696;887)	387	787	(682;878)	
9	375	802	(693;908)	396	792	(699;903)	
12	338	870	(750;988)	418	862	(747;978)	
		EPL intake (kcal/d)					
1		10	(5;16)				
2		14	(8;22)				
3		15	(9;27)				
4		21	(13;34)				
5		27	(16;47)				
6		28	(16;50)				
7		30	(17;51)				
8		31	(18;59)				
9		37	(19;66)				
12		46	(25;72)				
		Formula milk intake (kcal/d)			Formula milk intake (kcal/d)		
1		517	(435;576)		513	(443;574)	
2		537	(467;599)		544	(487;616)	*
3		545	(484;608)		574	(520;640)	*
4		563	(489;625)		591	(530;654)	*
5		506	(427;601)		562	(474;640)	*
6		463	(381;537)		468	(365;548)	
7		368	(305;471)		358	(290;458)	
8		350	(273;459)		340	(261;429)	
9		334	(252;432)		334	(259;392)	
12		272	(167;361)		256	(167;344)	
		Solids intake (kcal/d)			Solids intake (kcal/d)		
1		-	-		-	-	
2		-	-		-	-	
3		-	-		-	-	
4		0	(0;43)		0	(0;22)	*
5		110	(52;175)		65	(0;146)	*
6		195	(121;267)		207	(116;309)	
7		305	(211;421)		363	(231;482)	*
8		366	(269;486)		426	(324;534)	*
9		403	(293;526)		465	(361;576)	*
12		536	(422;688)		607	(478;733)	*

[a] Comparison was done with the Wilcoxon rank-sum test (* $p<0.05$)

Table S1: Percentage (%) and standard error (SE) of breastfed infants with consumption of instant tea, fruit juice or vegetable juice by country during the first year of life

		Age (completed months)					
		1	3	4	6	9	12
Germany	N	71	64	61	59	55	50
Belgium	N	23	27	37	48	44	46
Italy	N	147	127	117	112	99	102
Poland	N	28	48	45	44	41	41
Spain	N	80	71	70	58	46	48
Instant tea		1	3 [a]	4	6 [b]	9 [b]	12 [b]
				% (SE)			
Germany		4.2 (2.4)	1.6 (1.6)	1.6 (1.6)	3.4 (2.4)	3.6 (2.5)	10.0 (4.3)
Belgium		-	3.7 (3.7)	2.7 (2.7)	-	-	-
Italy		8.2 (2.3)	14.3 (3.1)	9.4 (2.7)	22.3 (4.0)	28.3 (4.5)	23.8 (4.2)
Poland		14.3 (6.7)	20.8 (5.9)	13.3 (5.1)	27.3 (6.8)	48.8 (7.9)	56.1 (7.8)
Spain		8.7 (3.2)	7.0 (3.1)	7.1 (3.1)	3.4 (2.4)	2.2 (2.2)	-
Fruit juice		1	3	4 [b]	6 [b]	9 [b]	12 [b]
Germany		-	-	1.6 (1.6)	16.9 (4.9)	38.2 (6.6)	58.0 (7.0)
Belgium		-	-	13.5 (5.6)	29.2 (6.6)	36.3 (7.3)	41.3 (7.3)
Italy		-	-	-	12.5 (3.1)	24.2 (4.3)	29.4 (4.5)
Poland		-	2.1 (2.0)	4.4 (3.1)	34.1 (7.2)	65.9 (7.5)	63.4 (7.6)
Spain		1.3 (1.3)	-	22.9 (5.1)	53.4 (6.6)	50.0 (7.4)	43.8 (7.2)
Vegetable juice		1	3	4	6 [b]	9 [b]	12 [b]
Germany		-	-	-	6.8 (3.3)	3.6 (2.5)	6.0 (3.4)
Belgium		-	-	-	2.1 (2.1)	-	-
Italy		-	-	-	-	-	-
Poland		-	-	-	15.9 (5.5)	36.6 (7.6)	31.7 (7.4)
Spain		-	-	-	-	-	-

Table S2: Percentage (%) and standard error (SE) of formula fed infants with consumption of instant tea, fruit juice or vegetable juice, by country during the first year

		Age (month completed)					
		1	3	4	6	9	12
Germany	N	116	139	131	126	109	101
Belgium	N	95	95	90	84	74	67
Italy	N	194	207	200	200	183	180
Poland	N	64	162	154	150	129	132
Spain	N	227	244	231	220	187	178

Instant tea	1	3 [a]	4	6 [b]	9 [b]	12 [b]
			% (SE)			
Germany	28.4 (4.2)	32.4 (4.0)	29.8 (4.0)	27.2 (4.0)	33.9 (4.6)	20.8 (4.1)
Belgium	1.1 (1.1)	2.1 (1.5)	1.1 (1.1)	2.4 (1.7)	2.7 (1.9)	1.5 (1.5)
Italy	24.7 (3.1)	26.6 (3.1)	31.5 (3.3)	31.3 (3.3)	22.4 (3.1)	19.4 (3.0)
Poland	87.5 (4.2)	80.9 (3.1)	75.3 (3.5)	74.0 (3.6)	72.1 (4.0)	71.2 (4.0)
Spain	25.6 (2.9)	14.8 (2.3)	12.6 (2.2)	6.4 (1.6)	1.6 (0.9)	1.1 (0.8)

Fruit juice	1	3	4 [b]	6 [b]	9 [b]	12 [b]
Germany	1.7 (1.2)	2.9 (1.4)	9.9 (2.6)	38.4 (4.3)	53.2 (4.8)	55.4 (5.0)
Belgium	-	2.1 1.5	11.1 (3.3)	39.2 (5.4)	44.5 (5.8)	34.3 (5.8)
Italy	-	-	2.0 (1.0)	9.7 (2.1)	23.0 (3.1)	29.4 (3.4)
Poland	-	0.1 (0.9)	19.4 (3.2)	47.3 (4.1)	67.4 (4.1)	70.4 (4.0)
Spain	2.2 (1.0)	7.8 (1.7)	23.8 (2.8)	53.6 (3.4)	49.7 (3.7)	39.3 (3.7)

Vegetable juice	1	3	4	6 [b]	9 [b]	12 [b]
Germany	-	-	5.3 (2.0)	5.6 (2.0)	4.6 (0.0)	4.0 (0.0)
Belgium	-	-	-	1.2 (1.2)	2.7 (1.9)	1.5 (1.5)
Italy	-	-	-	-	-	1.7 (1.0)
Poland	-	0.2 (0.1)	18.2 (3.1)	40.4 (4.0)	32.6 (4.1)	35.6 (4.2)
Spain	-	-	0.4 (0.4)	0.5 (0.5)	0.5 (0.5)	0.6 (0.6)

[a] $p<0.05$ [b] $p<0.001$

Table S3: Intake of energy providing liquids (EPL, ml/d) as well as formula milk (ml/d) by formula fed infants with and without EPL during the first year of life

Age (completed months)	N	Intake of EPL (ml/d)		Intake of formula milk with EPL (ml/d)		Intake of formula milk without EPL (ml/d)		p value
		(median)	(IQD)	(median)	(IQD)	(median)	(IQD)	
1	181	40	(10, 85)	738.3	(622, 825)	734.4	(635, 822)	
2	275	66	(30, 118)	770.0	(668, 868)	780.0	(698, 880)	*
3	277	73	(40, 133)	780.0	(693, 870)	821.7	(7, 16)	*
4	330	90	(45, 150)	803.4	(697, 894)	845.0	(757, 933)	*
5	384	80	(45, 160)	715.0	(600, 843)	799.4	(672, 900)	*
6	430	83	(40, 153)	642.3	(529, 747)	645.7	(516, 770)	
7	394	92	(46, 150)	506.7	(420, 650)	493.3	(400, 637)	
8	371	100	(47, 162)	483.3	(380, 632)	469.1	(359, 590)	
9	375	110	(50, 190)	463.3	(350, 600)	460.0	(357, 540)	
12	308	125	(73, 218)	400.0	(283, 527)	397.7	(280, 490)	

* p<0.05

Introduction of potentially allergenic foods in the infant´s diet during the first year of life in five European countries

Sonia A. Schiess[1], Veit Grote[2], Silvia Scaglioni[3], Veronica Luque[4], Francoise Martin[5], Anna Stolarczyk[6], Fiammetta Vecchi[3], Berthold Koletzko[1] (✉), for the European Childhood Obesity Project *

[1]Div. Metabolic Diseases & Nutrition, Dr. von Hauner Children's Hospital, Ludwig-Maximilian University, Munich, Germany, [2] Dept. Epidemiology, Inst. of Social Pediatrics and Adolescent Medicine, Ludwig-Maximilian University, Munich, Germany [3]Dept. of Pediatrics, San Paolo Hospital, Milan, Italy, [4]Pediatrics Research Unit, University Rovira i Virgili, Reus, Spain, [5]CHC St. Vincent, Rocourt, Belgium, [6]Clinic of Pediatrics, Children's Memorial Health Institute, Warsaw, Poland

*Study team:
Belgium (ULB Bruxelles and CHC St Vincent Liège): Carlier C, Goyens P, Hoyos J, Langhendries J-P, Van Hees J-N, Xhonneux A; **Germany** (Division of Pediatric Epidemiology, Institute of Social Pediatrics and Adolescent Medicine and Division of Nutritional Medicine and Metabolism, Dr. von Hauner Children's Hospital, Ludwig Maximilians University of Munich): Beyer J, Demmelmair H, Fritsch M, Handel U, Hannibal I, Kreichauf S, von Kries R, Pawellek I, Verwied-Jorky S; **Italy** (University of Milan): Giovannini M, Agostoni C, Confalonieri F, Tedeschi S, Vecchi F, Verduci E; **Spain** (Universitat Rovira i Virgili): Closa Monasterolo R, Escribano Subias J, Méndez Riera G; **Poland** (Children's Memorial Health Institute): Socha J, Dobrzańska A, Gruszfeld D, Socha P, Janas R, Pietraszek E, Kowalik A

Published in: Annals of Nutrition & Metabolism 2011;58:109-117; www.karger.com/anm

Abstract

Background: Little information is available on the ages of introducing potentially allergenic foods as part of complementary feeding. We aimed to analyze the age of introduction of potentially allergenic foods in healthy term infants relative to recommendations in 5 European countries.

Method: Recruitment was conducted from October 2002 to June 2004. A total of 1,678 infants [588 breastfed infants (BF) and 1,090 formula-fed infants (FF)] were studied. In 1,368 infants, at least one 3-day weighed food diary at the age of 1-9 and 12 completed months was available.

Results: Six percent of BF infants and 13% of FF infants consumed some potentially allergenic food already prior to the recommended minimum age of 4 months, and 4% of BF infants and 11% of FF infants had already received gluten. There were significant differences in the introduction of potentially allergenic foods between the countries at the age of 4-6 months ($p < 0.001$).

Conclusion: The time of first introduction of potentially allergenic foods in infants differed significantly between countries, and they were introduced much earlier than recommended in some countries. FF infants received potentially allergenic foods earlier than BF infants. Better information and counseling of parents is desirable.

Introduction

Allergic manifestations in children have increased in both western and developing countries.(1) Diet in infancy may have an effect on health throughout childhood and adulthood, including the manifestation of atopic diseases.(1-6)

In 2001, the World Health Organization (WHO) issued a revised global recommendation that infants should be exclusively breastfed during the first 6 months of life before any complementary food is introduced.(7) There were no specific guidelines for the introduction of complementary foods known as potentially allergenic foods, neither for healthy infants nor for infants with risk of atopic diseases. Complementary foods like cow's milk, cereal with gluten, hen's egg, fish, nuts or soy bean are considered potentially allergenic foods.(8;9)

Different studies have associated a very early introduction of complementary foods with an increased development of atopic diseases. Saarinen and Kajoosari (10) reported that breastfeeding for at least 6 months protected against atopic dermatitis throughout childhood and adolescence. Even though numerous observational studies have explored the potential impact of breast feeding on the development of allergies and eczema, the data remain controversial.(6) The most convincing data are available for benefits of breast feeding in infants at high risk with a first degree relative with atopic disease, in which two meta-analyses found a transient protective effect of exclusive breastfeeding for at least 4 months on later atopic dermatitis, wheezing and asthma in infancy and early childhood. (11;12)

In Australian infants, the introduction of milk other than breast milk before 4 months of age had a strong association with asthma and atopy in children at the age of 6 years.(13) Infants exposed to 4 or more different types of solid foods before the age of 4 months had a 2.9-fold higher risk of eczema up to the age of 10 years than those not exposed to early solid feeding.(4) Fiocchi et al. (14) suggested to introducing complementary feeding after the age of 6 months with caution and only one kind at a time, including potentially allergenic foods like egg, peanut, nuts and fish. A review of the European Academy of Allergology and Clinical Immunology concluded that the most effective dietary measure for the prevention of atopic diseases even in high-risk patients is exclusive breastfeeding until preferably 6 months, but at least for 4 completed months with avoidance of solid foods and cows' milk in that time period.(9;15) However, recent studies showed delayed introduction of complementary foods associated with increased development of atopic disease.(1;16-21) The ESPGHAN Committee on Nutrition recently concluded that there is no convincing scientific evidence that avoidance, or delayed introduction after the beginning of the 7th month of age, of potentially allergenic foods, such as fish and eggs, reduces allergies. (5) Here, we describe the practice of introducing potentially allergenic foods as part of complementary feeding in apparently healthy term infants in 5 European countries participating in the European Childhood Obesity Project, including countries of central, west, east and south (Mediterranean) Europe with different traditions and eating behaviors.

Subjects and Methods
Study Design

It was our aim to analyze the consumption of potentially allergenic foods as part of complementary feeding versus recommendations in apparently healthy infants. Data were collected as part of the EU Childhood Obesity Project (22;23). In brief, recruitment of healthy infants born at term occurred between the 1 October 2002 and the 31 July 2004 in 11 study centers in Germany (Munich and Nuremberg), Belgium (Brussels and Liège), Italy (Milano), Spain (Tarragona and Reus) and Poland (Warsaw).

Invited for the study were healthy, singleton, term infants with mothers ≥18 years, with good knowledge of the national language and residence in the area of the respective study center. Exclusion criteria were mothers with hormonal or metabolic diseases or illicit addiction during pregnancy (22). Mothers were approached by study personnel at the maternity hospitals before their discharge or via pediatricians and midwifes. After oral information and written consent, mothers and infants were invited for an initial medical visit with collection of anthropometric measurements and socio-demographic data as well as of data about the medical history of infants and parents including a history of allergy and atopic diseases, pregnancy and delivery. In the following months, parents and infants were followed up regularly with visits in the study centers and mailed questionnaires, including 3-day weighed food diaries at the age of 1-9 and 12 months.

Study Population

The study group comprised 2 double-blind randomized groups of FF infants with different protein levels and 1 reference group of BF infants (22). BF infants had to be exclusively breastfed for at least 3 complete months, and FF infants were randomized to one of the study formula milks before the age of 8 weeks.

Data Collection

Anthropometric data and data from standardized questionnaires were introduced at each study center and transferred into a central data base (RDE Software GmbH, Munich, Germany). At the age of 1-9 and 12 months, parents were asked to complete a 3-day food protocol (including 2 weekdays and 1 weekend day). The dietary data were collected prospectively, and no attempts were made to modify parental decision making on introducing solids, liquids or potentially allergenic foods to the infant diet. The study personnel were explicitly advised to collect detailed information on dietary intake of the infants and to provide no recommendations on complementary feeding to the parents. The food protocol data were introduced into our own software by nutritionists at the different study centers and then transferred into a central data base. Standard operating procedures were developed to harmonize the calculation and introduction of food intake data.

At the beginning of the study, mothers and fathers were asked about their history of allergy and atopic diseases like a doctor's diagnosis of asthma, hay fever, allergy, atopic dermatitis or others.

Allergenic Foods

Complementary foods consumed during the first year of life by the infants of all 5 countries (3,281 food items) were classified by their ingredients. We defined as potentially allergenic complementary foods any foods containing gluten, milk, egg, fish, soy or nuts. For the evaluation of milk introduction, we included any milk or dairy product other than infant or follow-on formula. This included primarily cow's milk and products derived from cow's milk and, in a few cases, milk from goat, sheep or buffalo and their products.

We defined as soy product any food item containing soy (e.g., soy milk, soy yogurt, lecithin of soy, soybean oil) and as soy protein any food item containing soy protein (e.g., soy milk, soy formula, soy yogurt, tofu, dessert from soy milk).

Sociodemographic Data

We grouped mothers into 4 categories based on age at delivery: category I = age ≤25 years; category II = age >25 to 30 years; category III = age >30 to 35 years, and category IV = age >35 years. Maternal educational levels were categorized in 3 groups: no/low education = pre-preliminary to lower secondary (no schooling to elementary education); middle education = upper secondary and post-secondary (high school), and high education = first and second stage of tertiary education (college, university or institutes of technology).

Statistics

To avoid cofounders, we decided to analyze BF and FF infants in separate groups. Mainly the χ^2 test and logistic regression analysis were used to investigate differences in the introduction of potentially allergenic foods. Stata 9.2, SPSS 16.0, and Excel were used for data analyses.

Ethics

The study protocol was reviewed by the ethic committees of all study centers. Written informed parental consent was obtained for each infant.

Results

A total of 1,678 infants, 588 BF and 1090 FF infants, and their mothers/parents were recruited and their data analyzed. At least one 3-day food diary was available for evaluation in 1,368 (82%) infants. At the age of 3 completed months, 1,183 3-day weighed food diaries could be evaluated, at 4 completed months 1,135, at 6 completed months 1,074, at 9 completed months 966, and at 12 completed months 944 (table 1). At the age of 2 and 3 months, we analyzed the food protocols from 95% (1,127/1,184) of all infants in the study, from 77% (983/1,275) between the age of 3 and 6 months, from 72% (808/1,116) between 3 and 9 months, and from 70% (756/1,085) up to 12 months of age. Some sociodemographic characteristics of the study BF and FF infants are shown in table S1.

BF Infants

In our study population, 92% of the BF infants were breastfed until the age of 20 weeks and 75% until the age of 28 weeks.

At the age of 4 completed months, we found some 6% of BF infants consuming at least one potentially allergenic food and 51% at the age of 6 completed months (fig. 1). The median for the introduction of potentially allergenic food was at the age of 28 weeks (95% CI 27.3-28.7) for BF infants.

Data from the food protocols showed no BF infant with an intake of food with gluten at the age of 3 completed months, while 4% of BF infants received food with gluten at the age of 4 completed months and 32% at the age of 6 completed months (fig. 1).

We found significant differences between the countries in the proportions of BF infants with intake of food with gluten (at each month at the ages of 4-9 months; p < 0.001; table 2). At the age of 4 completed months, 22% of the BF infants in Belgium, 6% in Spain and 2% in Italy consumed some food with gluten. At the age of 6 completed months, we found the highest proportion of BF infants with an intake of food with gluten in Belgium (58%)

and the lowest in Poland (7%) (table 2). After comparing several parameters of the parents of BF infants receiving gluten before the national recommended time point of introduction, we found the lowest proportion of BF infants receiving gluten by mothers with the lowest educational level ($p < 0.05$).

At the age of 4 and 6 completed months, 3 and 39% of the BF infants, respectively, consumed some milk or food with milk or milk product other than breast milk or formula milk (fig. 1). We found significant differences in the percentages of infants with consumption of milk or milk products between the countries in each month at the age of 4-12 months ($p < 0.01$; table 2). At the ages of 4 and 5 completed months, we found the highest proportions of BF infants with an intake of milk or food with milk or milk product in Belgium (19 and 22%, respectively; table 2). In the second half of the first year, Italy had the highest proportion of BF infants with milk or food with milk or milk product consumption (77-99%). In contrast, we found the lowest proportions of infants with an intake of milk or food with milk or milk product at the age of 6-9 months in Poland (0-59%) and in Germany (20-56%).

Some 1 and 4% of the BF infants consumed some egg or food with egg at the ages of 4 and 6 months, respectively (Fig. 1). The time points for introduction of egg or food with egg were significantly different between the countries (at each month from 4 to 12 months; $p < 0.005$; table 2). At the age of 4 and 5 completed months, only infants in Belgium received some egg or food with egg (5 and 7%, respectively) and at the age of 6 completed months they had the highest proportion of infants with consumption of egg or food with egg (21%), while in the other countries, not more than 2% of all BF infants consumed some egg or food with egg. At the age of 7-12 completed months, Poland (30-76%), Belgium (29-76%) and Germany (10-62%) had the highest proportions of infants with egg or food with egg intake, whereas in Italy and Spain, no more than 10% of the BF infants had received some egg or food with egg until the age of 9 months.

No fish or food with fish was eaten until the age of 4 completed months, and only 2% of all BF infants received fish or food with fish at the age of 6 completed months (fig. 1). Separated by country, 6% in Belgium, 4% in Spain and 2% in Italy consumed some fish or food with fish at the age of 6 completed months (table 2). At the age of 7-12 completed months, Italy (17-71%), Belgium (15-48%) and Spain (4-73%) had the highest proportions of infants with fish or food with fish intake. In Germany and Poland, no more than 10% of the infants consumed fish or food with fish during the first year of life.

Nuts or some food with nuts were consumed by <4 and 8% of the BF infants at the ages of

9 and 12 months, respectively. During the first year of life, we found the highest proportions of infants with nut or food with nut intake in Belgium (17%) and Germany (14%) and the lowest in Italy (3%), Poland (5%) and Spain (4%).

Many infants in Belgium (up to 54%) and Germany (up to 37%) consumed soy products or food with soy during the first year of life, whereas in the other countries, no more than 5% of the BF infants consumed soy products or food with soy. However, not more than 4% of the BF infants consumed soy protein or food with soy protein (soy formula milk, soy milk dessert, ingredient of a dish) during the first year. There were very low proportions of infants with an intake of food with soy protein (fig. 1). In Italy, we found 1-3% of the BF infants with intake of food with soy protein from the age of 4-12 months, and we found the highest proportion in Belgium with up to 11% (table 2).

We found significant differences in sociodemographic characteristics (table S1) between the study groups of each country in BF infants, but there was no association between intake of food with gluten, milk, egg and fish and maternal age at birth, educational level and smoking habit, nor with the infant's birth weight and birth order of the infants.

About 31% of the BF infants had a parent with a history of allergy and atopic diseases (18% of the fathers, 16% of the mothers) at the beginning of the study. There were no significant differences in the proportions of mothers, fathers or both parents with a history of allergy and atopic diseases between the countries.

FF Infants

In our study cohort, 249 (23%) infants were exclusively formula fed since birth, all others gradually switched from breastfeeding to formula feeding within the first 8 weeks of life. The median age was 14 days (interquartile range 3-30) at randomization and 16 days (interquartile range 2-29) at the baseline visit.

Some 13% of FF infants consumed at least one potentially allergenic food at the age of 4 completed months and 59% at the age of 6 completed months (fig. 1). The median for the introduction of potentially allergenic food was at the age of 26 weeks (95% CI 25.2-26.2) for FF infants. It was significantly earlier compared to the BF infants (p < 0.001).

We found 0.3% FF infants with consumption of food with gluten at the age of 1 month, 0.8% at 2, 2% at 3 and 11% at the age of 4 completed months. At the age of 6 completed months, 43% of the FF infants consumed some food with gluten (fig. 1).

There were significant differences between countries in the proportions of FF infants with consumption of products containing gluten in each one of the first 9 months of life (p <

0.001; table 3). Belgium had the highest proportions of infants with an intake of food with gluten in the first 5 completed months of life (up to 38%). At the age of 4 completed months in Belgium, Germany and Italy, more than 10-25% of FF infants had been fed some food with gluten. At 6 completed months, Germany (70%) had the highest and Poland (27%) and Spain (28%) the lowest proportions of FF infants with food intake with gluten.

Milk or any food with milk or dairy product other than infant formula was consumed at the ages of 4 and 6 completed months by 7 and 44% of the FF infants, respectively (fig. 1). The proportions of FF infants with intake of milk, food with milk or dairy products were significantly different between the countries (in each month, 2-12 months of age, $p < 0.05$). At the age of 2-4 completed months, Belgium had the highest proportions of infants with an intake of some milk other than formula milk (3-14%; table 3). At the age of 5-12 completed months, Germany (39-96%) and Italy (88-100%) had the highest proportion of infants with consumption of milk, food with milk or dairy products intake, Poland (5-93%) and Spain (7-91%) the lowest. In Italy, more than 90% of the FF infants had received some milk or dairy products at the age of 7 completed months.

At the age of 5-8 months, we found significantly higher proportions of FF infants with milk, food with milk or dairy products intake with a low and middle maternal educational level compared to infants of mothers with a higher educational level ($p < 0.05$).

Less than 1% of FF infants consumed some food with egg during the first 4 months of life, not more than 4% at the age of 6 completed months (fig. 1) and <10% in each country (table 3). In the second half of the first year, we found the highest proportions of FF infants with an intake of egg or some food with egg in Poland (43-90%), Belgium (8-64%) and Germany (8-73%), and the lowest in Italy (1-42%) and Spain (0-30%; table 3).

No infant consumed any fish or some food with fish until the age of 4 completed months and not more than 2% at the age of 6 completed months (fig. 1). Belgium (19-49%), Italy (17-56%) and Spain (8-74%) had the highest proportions of FF infants with fish or some food with fish intake during 7-12 months of age (table 3).

Nuts or some food with nuts were consumed by <7% of all FF infants during the first year of life. The highest proportions of infants with nut intake or of some food with nuts were in Belgium (22%; through Muesli, cookies, Nutella, pudding, syrup) and Germany (18%; through cakes or cookies, Muesli, Nutella, pudding, bread) and <3% in the other countries during the first year of life.

Some 2 and 6% of all FF infants consumed soy products or some food with soy products at the age of 4 and 6 completed months, respectively. At the age of 4 and 6 completed months, 1 and 10% of FF infants in Germany consumed soy products or some food with soy products, and 12 and 43% in Belgium. In the other countries, there was no consumption of food with soy products during the first 6 months of life.

Less than 1% of all FF infants consumed some food with soy protein (soy formula, tofu, dessert from soy milk) during the first year (fig. 1). FF infants receiving foods with soy protein during the first year of life were only found in Germany and Belgium (not more than 3%; table 3).

We found significant differences in sociodemographic characteristics (table S1) between the study groups of each country in FF infants but there were no associations between the intake of food with gluten, milk, egg and fish and birth weight, birth order or smoking habits of the mother.

About 21% of the FF infants had a parent with a history of allergy and atopic diseases (11% of the fathers, 13% of the mothers). We found significant different proportions of mothers ($p < 0.001$) and fathers ($p = 0.003$) with a history of allergy and atopic diseases between the countries.

Discussion

In our study population of apparently healthy infants, FF infants received potentially allergenic foods like foods with gluten, milk and egg earlier than BF infants. In contrast, soy protein was introduced earlier and in higher proportion to BF infants, mainly due to the introduction of soy formula. There were large differences between countries for the introduction of potentially allergenic foods.

Although European and national recommendations advised not to introduce complementary foods before 4 months (5;9) or even before 6 months of age (6), 6% of BF infants and 13% of FF infants had received potentially allergenic food (mainly foods with gluten and milk) at the age of 4 completed months. National recommendations at the time of our data collection advised to introduce foods with gluten not before 6 months and even from 8 months onwards in Spain and after the age of 9 months in Poland (24-27), congruent with the lowest proportion of BF and FF infants consuming gluten until the age of 9 months in these two countries.

Intake of foods containing gluten before the age of 3 months was associated with increased islet autoantibody in infants (28). The highest proportion of FF infants receiving foods with gluten was found in Belgium (10%) due to the consumption of flour mixtures, cereals for infant porridge and cookies. Traditionally, there is a high consumption of antireflux infant formula in Belgium which may have led to more frequent use of cereals in the infant diet during the first months of life.

The intake of milk or dairy products as separate food items or as ingredients of foods other than breast milk or formula milk were highest in Belgian BF infants at the age of 4 and 5 completed months and in Belgian FF infants at the age of 2-4 completed months due to the consumption of milk-cereal meals, cookies, dairy products or as ingredient of meals. From the age of 6 completed months, we find the highest proportions of infants with consumption of some milk in Italy, probably due to the use of milk porridge and cheese (Grana, Parmigiano, Formaggino) added to the infant's meal. Some 76% of BF infants and 84% of FF infants of the total cohort consumed any milk other than infant formula at the age of 9 completed months and around 95% at the age of 12 months. Thus, nearly all infants received cow's milk during the first year of life, mostly as part of a milk cereal meal, as milk product (yogurt, curd mixture or cheese) or as ingredient of a product or meal but not as drink. In most countries, the introduction of cow's milk as drink is recommended to be delayed until after 12 months of age (5).

The consumption of milk other than breast milk or infant or follow-on formula in apparently healthy infants, especially in FF infants consuming formula milk based on cow's milk, may be irrelevant with respect to the risk of atopy. Milk or dairy products were consumed at the ages of 4 and 6 completed months by 3 and 39% of BF infants and 6 and 44% of FF infants, respectively.

Almost no food with egg, fish and soy protein was consumed during the first 6 months by BF and FF infants. Around 52% of BF infants and 56% of FF infants consumed some egg or food with egg and 48% of BF and 44% of FF infants consumed some fish or food with fish at the end of the first year of life. Indeed, we found significant differences between the countries in the proportions of BF and FF infants with some consumption of egg or fish during the second half of the year. The highest proportion of infants with fish intake was found in Italy, Belgium and Spain. This was in line with the national recommendations that suggested fish intake after 6 months in Belgium, not before 7-8 months in Italy, 9-10 months in Spain and not earlier than at the age of 2 years in Poland. When evaluating sociodemographic characteristics and the parental history of allergy and atopic diseases with regard to the time of potential allergenic food introduction in relation to the national recommendations of each country, separated by BF and FF infants, we found that the age of the mother, her educational level and the parental history of allergy and atopic diseases in some cases influenced the time point of introduction (data not shown). National eating habits and geographic distance of the study centers to the sea may further influence feeding practice.

The presence or absence of maternal allergy or atopic disease does not affect the consumption patterns of potentially allergenic foods during the first year of life (table S2). When applying multiple regression analysis for BF and FF infants for each month at the ages of 3-6 months, including the effects of maternal or paternal history of allergy or atopic diseases, country of residence, maternal age, maternal education level and smoking behavior, the strongest and most consistent predictor was the country of residence.

For our dietary data collection, we have chosen 3-day weighed food protocols, one of the most reliable methods for capturing eating habits of children. One limitation of this method is that foods which are not eaten on a regular basis may not be captured. Since food intake during the first months of life is relatively uniform, a 3-day food protocol is considered quite representative of infant eating habits. Also, there was a high percentage of infants with monthly food protocols (95% in the first months and 70% between 3 and 12 months of age).

In conclusion, this study documents an earlier introduction of potentially allergenic foods in FF infants than in BF infants as well as significant differences between countries for the time of introduction. Recent studies indicate that the introduction of complementary foods - including potentially allergenic foods - between the age of 4 and 6 completed months was associated with a reduced risk of food allergy and atopic diseases, in some observations with stronger protective effects if the infant was still breastfed at the time of complementary food introduction (1;15;29-31). These data support simplification of recommendations and practice of complementary feeding, with introduction of all suitable complementary foods in all infants not before 17 weeks and not later than 26 weeks of age (5).

Acknowledgements

We are very grateful to the families participating in this study, for the efforts and time they have invested, as well as to the collaborating physicians, midwifes and nurses for their helpful support in recruitment. We thank the whole study team for their effort, endurance and dedication to this work and for their help in informing and recruiting families. The European Childhood Obesity Project is being carried out with financial support of the European Community, under the 5th Framework Programme for Research, Technology and Demonstration 'Quality of Life and Management of Living Resources', Key Action 1

(Food, Nutrition and Health), contract number QLK1-CT2002-389, and the 6th Framework Priority 5.4.3.1 Food Quality and Safety (Early Nutrition Programming - long term follow-up of efficacy and safety trials and integrated epidemiological, genetic, animal, consumer and economic research, EARNEST, Food-CT-2005-007036).

Berthold Koletzko is the recipient of a Freedom to Discover Award of the Bristol Myers Squibb Foundation, New York, N.Y., USA. The presented data are part of the PhD Thesis in Human Biology submitted by Sonia A. Schiess to the Medical Faculty of Ludwig Maximilian University of Munich.

Reference List

1. Greer FR, Sicherer SH, Burks AW, and the Committee on Nutrition and Section on Allergy and Immunology. Effects of Early Nutritional Interventions on the Development of Atopic Disease in Infants and Children: The Role of Maternal Dietary Restriction, Breastfeeding, Timing of Introduction of Complementary Foods, and Hydrolyzed Formulas. Pediatrics 2008;121:183-91.
2. Foote KD, Marriott LD. Weaning of infants. Arch Dis Child 2003;88:488-92.
3. Kajosaari M. Atopy prevention in childhood: the role of diet. Pediatr Allergy Immunol 1994;5 (Suppl):26-8.
4. Fergusson DM, Horwood LJ, Shannon FT. Early Solid Feeding and Recurrent Childhood Eczema: A 10-Year Longitudinal Study. Pediatrics 1990;86:541-6.
5. ESPGHAN Committee of Nutrition: Agostoni C, Decsi T, Fewtrell M et al. Complementary feeding: a commentary by the ESPGHAN Committee on Nutrition. J Pediatr Gastroenterol Nutr 2008;46:99-110.
6. ESPGHAN Committee on Nutrition:, Agostoni C, Braegger C et al. Breast-feeding: A Commentary by the ESPGHAN Committee on Nutrition. J Pediatr Gastroenterol Nutr 2009;49:112-25.
7. WHO 54th World Health Assembly. Infant and young child nutrition. WHA54.2. 2001.
8. Koletzko B. Complementary Foods and the Development of Food Allergy. Pediatrics 2000;106(5):1285.
9. Host A, Koletzko B, Dreborg S et al. Dietary products used in infants for treatment and prevention of food allergy. Joint statement of the European Society for Paediatric Allergology and Clinical Immunology (ESPACI) Committee on

Hypoallergenic Formulas and the European Society for Paediatric Gastroenterology, Hepatology and Nutrition (ESPGHAN) Committee on Nutrition. Arch Dis Child 1999;81:80-4.

10. Saarinen UM, Kajosaari M. Breastfeeding as prophylaxis against atopic disease: prospective follow-up study until 17 years old. The Lancet 1995;346:1065-9.

11. Van Rossum CMT Buechner FI, Hoechstra J. Quantification of health effects of breastfeeding. Dutch State Institute for Nutrition and Health 2005.Dutch State Institute for Nutrition and Health. RIVM Report 350040001/2005. http://www.rivm.nl/bibliotheek/rapporten/350040001.pdf.

12. Agency for Healthcare Research and Quality. Breastfeeding and maternal and infant health outcomes in developed countries. AHRQ publication No 07-E007 2007 2007;Dutch State Institute for Nutrition and Health. www.ncbi.nlm.nih.gov/books/bv.fcgi?rid=hstat1b.chapter.106732.

13. Oddy WH, Holt PG, Sly PD et al. Association between breast feeding and asthma in 6 year old children: findings of a prospective birth cohort study. BMJ 1999;319:815-9.

14. Fiocchi A, Assa'ad A, Bahna S. Food allergy and the introduction of solid foods to infants: a consensus document. Annals of Allergy, Asthma and Immunology 2006;97:10-21.

15. Muraro A, Dreborg S, Halken S et al. Dietary prevention of allergic diseases in infants and small children. Part III: Critical review of published peer-reviewed observational and interventional studies and final recommendations. Pediatr Allergy Immunol 2004;15:291-307.

16. Zutavern A, Brockow I, Schaaf B et al. Timing of Solid Food Introduction in Relation to Atopic Dermatitis and Atopic Sensitization: Results From a Prospective Birth Cohort Study. Pediatrics 2006;117:401-11.

17. Zutavern A, Brockow I, Schaaf B et al. Timing of solid food introduction in relation to eczema, asthma, allergic rhinitis, and food and inhalant sensitization at the age of 6 years: results from the prospective birth cohort study LISA. Pediatrics 2008;121:e44-e52.

18. Filipiak B, Zutavern A, Koletzko S et al. Solid Food Introduction in Relation to Eczema: Results from a Four-Year Prospective Birth Cohort Study. The Journal of Pediatrics 2007;151:352-8.

19. Snijders BEP, Thijs C, van Ree R, van den Brandt PA. Age at First Introduction of Cow Milk Products and Other Food Products in Relation to Infant Atopic Manifestations in the First 2 Years of Life: The KOALA Birth Cohort Study. Pediatrics 2008;122:e115-e122.
20. Alm B, Aberg N, Erdes L et al. Early introduction of fish decreases the risk of eczema in infants. Arch Dis Child 2009;94:11-5.
21. Kull I, Bergström A, Lilja G, Pershagen G, Wickman M. Fish consumption during the first year of life and development of allergic diseases during childhood. Allergy 2006;61:1009-15.
22. Koletzko B, von Kries R, Monasterolo RC et al. Lower protein in infant formula is associated with lower weight up to age 2 years: a randomized clinical trial. Am J Clin Nutr 2009;89:1-10.
23. Schiess S, Grote V, Scaglioni S et al. Introduction of complementary feeding in five European countries. J Pediatr Gastroenterol Nutr 2010;50(1):92-8.
24. O.N.E. Bon appétit les bébés ! Fernand Gaubelle (Ed). O.N.E. Pamphlet 1998; 20-39.
25. Savino, F., Castagno, E., and Silvestro, L. Lo Svezzamento: La Realtà pratica. Milano Pediatria 2004 .
26. Ksiazyk J, Rudzka-Kantoch Z, Weker H. Feeding plan for breast-fed infants and non-breast-fed infants. Medycyna Praktyczna Pediatria 2001;5:1-2.
27. Lázaro Almarza A. Diversificación alimentaria en pediatría. An Esp Pediatr 2001;54:150-2.
28. Ziegler A-G, Schmid S, Huber D, Hummel M, Bonifacio E. Early Infant Feeding and Risk of Developing Type 1 Diabetes-Associated Autoantibodies. JAMA 2003;290:1721-8.
29. Ivarsson A, Hernell O, Stenlund H, Persson LA. Breast-feeding protects against celiac disease. Am J Clin Nutr 2002;75:914-21.
30. Akobeng AK, Ramanan AV, Buchan I, Heller RF. Effect of breast feeding on risk of celiac disease: a systematic review and meta-analysis of observational studies. Arch Dis Child 2006;91:39-43.
31. Norris JM, Barriga K, Hoffenberg EJ et al. Risk of Celiac Disease Autoimmunity and Timing of Gluten Introduction in the Diet of Infants at Increased Risk of Disease. JAMA 2005;293:2343-51.

Table 1: Number of infants and percentages by country of evaluated 3-day food protocols at the age of 4, 6, 9 and 12 months

	Age (completed months)									
	3		4		6		9		12	
	n	%	n	%	n	%	n	%	n	%
BF infants										
Germany	64	19	61	19	59	19	55	19	50	17
Belgium	27	8	37	11	48	15	44	15	46	16
Italy	126	38	116	35	109	34	98	35	101	35
Poland	48	14	45	14	44	14	41	14	41	14
Spain	71	21	70	21	57	18	46	16	48	17
Total	336	100	329	100	317	100	284	100	286	100
FF infants										
Germany	139	16	131	16	125	17	109	16	101	15
Belgium	95	11	90	11	80	11	74	11	67	10
Italy	207	24	200	25	193	25	183	27	180	27
Poland	162	19	154	19	146	19	129	19	132	20
Spain	244	29	231	29	213	28	187	27	178	27
Total	847	100	806	100	757	100	682	100	658	100

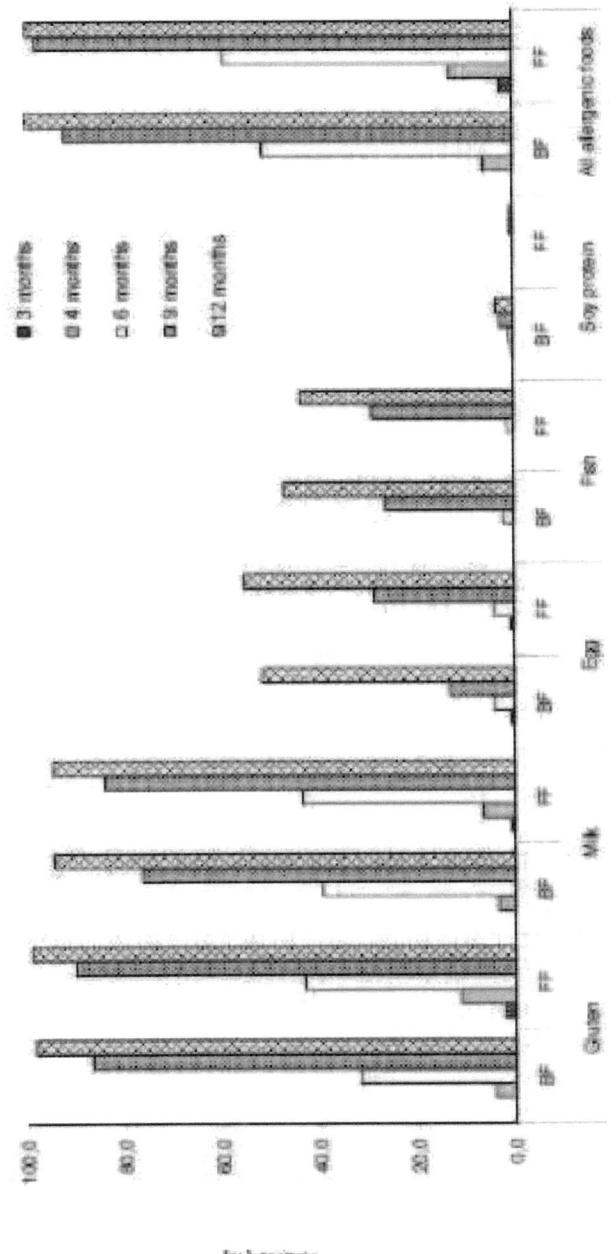

Figure 1: Percentage (%) of BF and FF infants with intake of potentially allergenic foods during the first year

Table 2: Percentage (%) of breast fed infants with intake of typical allergenic foods at the age of 4, 6, 9 and 12 months

	Age (completed month)			
Gluten	4 [a]	6 [a]	9 [b]	12
Germany	-	28.8	85.5	100.0
Belgium	21.6	58.3	90.9	97.8
Italy	1.7	34.9	94.9	100.0
Poland	-	6.8	75.6	92.7
Spain	5.7	26.3	76.1	97.9
Milk	4 [b]	6 [a]	9 [a]	12 [b]
Germany	-	20.3	56.4	84.0
Belgium	18.9	43.8	75.0	95.7
Italy	1.7	77.1	96.9	99.0
Poland	-	-	58.5	95.1
Spain	2.9	14.0	73.9	93.8
Egg	4 [b]	6 [a]	9 [a]	12 [a]
Germany	-	1.7	18.2	62.0
Belgium	5.4	20.8	43.2	76.1
Italy	-	0.9	10.2	32.7
Poland	-	2.3	53.7	75.6
Spain	-	-	8.7	37.5
Fish	4	6	9 [a]	12 [a]
Germany	-	-	1.8	10.0
Belgium	-	6.3	25.0	47.8
Italy	-	1.8	52.0	71.3
Poland	-	-	-	2.4
Spain	-	3.5	26.1	72.9
Soy protein	4	6	9	12 [c]
Germany	-	-	-	2.0
Belgium	-	-	6.8	10.9
Italy	0.9	2.8	3.1	3.0
Poland	-	-	4.9	2.4
Spain	-	-	-	-

Applying χ^2 test for each month of age, we found significant differences ([a] $p<0.001$ [b] $p<0.01$ [c] $p<0.05$) in the proportions of BF infants with intake of potentially allergenic foods like (gluten, milk, egg, fish and soy protein) between the countries.

Table 3: Percentage (%) of formula fed infants with intake of typical allergenic foods at the age of 4, 6, 9 and 12 month

	Age (completed months)			
	4 [a]	6 [a]	9 [a]	12
Gluten				
Germany	13.7	69.6	97.2	99.0
Belgium	24.4	51.3	97.3	98.5
Italy	10.5	51.3	96.7	99.4
Poland	5.2	26.7	81.4	98.5
Spain	9.1	28.2	85.6	98.9
Milk	4 [a]	6 [a]	9 [b]	12 [a]
Germany	11.5	58.4	92.7	96.0
Belgium	14.4	31.3	79.7	91.0
Italy	9.5	87.6	97.3	100.0
Poland	0.6	15.8	72.1	93.2
Spain	1.7	18.8	75.9	91.0
Egg	4	6 [a]	9 [a]	12 [a]
Germany	2.3	8.0	32.1	73.3
Belgium	1.1	7.5	59.5	64.2
Italy	0.5	0.5	9.3	41.7
Poland	-	9.6	65.9	90.2
Spain	-	-	8.0	30.3
Fish	4	6 [c]	9 [a]	12 [a]
Germany	-	-	5.5	8.9
Belgium	-	3.8	40.5	49.3
Italy	-	2.6	45.9	55.6
Poland	-	-	2.3	11.4
Spain	-	0.9	40.1	73.6
Soy protein	4	6	9	12 [b]
Germany	-	-	1.8	3.0
Belgium	1.1	1.3	2.7	3.0
Italy	-	-	-	-
Poland	-	-	-	-
Spain	-	-	0.5	-

Applying χ^2 test for each month of age, we found significant differences ([a] $p<0.001$ [b] $p<0.01$ [c] $p<0.05$) in the proportions of FF infants with intake of potentially allergenic foods like (gluten, milk, egg, fish and soy protein) between the countries.

Table S1: Sociodemographic characteristics of BF infant and FF infants

		BF infants						FF infants					
		Germany %	Belgium %	Italy %	Poland %	Spain %	p value	Germany %	Belgium %	Italy %	Poland %	Spain %	p value
Mothers age (years)	≤25	7.6	17.6	4.2	6.4	7.6	<0.001	17.5	16.1	4.7	42.3	11.0	<0.001
	>25 to 30	15.9	35.8	21.1	62.7	18.2		33.1	34.6	28.1	34.5	33.3	
	>30 to 35	42.6	36.6	48.7	21.4	50.2		33.7	39.0	35.5	17.6	37.1	
	>35	33.9	10.0	26.0	9.5	24.0		15.6	10.2	31.8	5.6	18.6	
Foreign parents	yes	2.3	12.8	3.0	0.0	3.5	<0.001	11.7	2.5	5.5	0.0	0.9	<0.001
Mothers educational level	low	4.8	5.6	12.6	1.7	15.6	<0.001	30.4	12.4	30.3	24.7	37.3	<0.001
	middle	40.7	43.5	63.8	35.2	33.1		58.6	54.6	57.3	51.1	46.9	
	high	54.5	50.9	23.6	63.2	51.3		11.0	32.9	12.4	24.2	15.8	
Fathers educational level	low	0.0	9.3	24.0	1.9	22.3	<0.001	26.0	10.6	35.1	26.7	45.3	<0.001
	middle	27.4	39.2	59.4	42.5	37.1		54.7	60.6	51.0	61.0	43.6	
	high	72.6	51.5	16.6	55.6	40.6		19.2	28.8	13.9	12.2	11.1	
Household size	2 members	1.8	2.0	0.0	0.0	0.0	<0.001	6.9	2.4	0.0	0.0	1.4	<0.001
	3 members	56.4	55.5	59.8	57.7	55.6		51.0	48.2	57.7	37.6	50.4	
	4 members	29.1	32.7	29.8	18.1	32.9		27.2	27.0	32.9	27.0	37.1	
	>4 members	12.7	9.7	10.4	24.2	11.5		14.9	22.4	9.4	35.4	11.2	
Birth order	1st child	58.2	58.1	65.7	66.3	56.0	<0.001	55.8	50.6	59.6	62.7	52.5	<0.001
	2nd child	28.1	36.1	29.9	24.2	32.0		32.2	26.7	30.4	28.7	40.0	
	3rd child	12.1	3.6	4.4	9.5	7.0		9.0	18.3	6.9	6.2	6.9	
	>3 children	1.7	2.3	0.0	0.0	0.0		3.0	4.3	3.1	2.4	0.6	

Table S2: BF infants and FF infants of mothers with and without history of allergy or atopic diseases, with and without consumption of potentially allergenic foods, during the first year of life

Age (completed months)	Infants receiving potentially allergenic food	BF infants				FF infants			
		Mother with history of allergy or atopic diseases				Mother with history of allergy or atopic diseases			
		no		yes		no		yes	
		N	%	N	%	N	%	N	%
1	no	275	100,0%	72	98,6%	604	99,7%	87	100,0%
	yes	0	0%	1	1,4%	2	,3%	0	0%
2	no	268	99,7%	71	100,0%	731	98,8%	105	99,1%
	yes	1	,3%	0	0%	9	1,2%	1	,9%
3	no	269	99,3%	64	98,5%	723	97,3%	108	99,0%
	yes	2	,7%	1	1,5%	20	2,7%	1	1,0%
4	no	243	91,7%	60	93,8%	611	88,3%	83	84,7%
	yes	22	8,3%	4	6,3%	97	13,7%	15	15,3%
5	no	213	80,1%	45	69,2%	444	63,6%	57	58,2%
	yes	53	19,9%	20	30,8%	254	36,4%	41	41,8%
6	no	117	45,2%	30	51,7%	267	40,0%	30	33,7%
	yes	142	54,8%	28	48,3%	401	60,0%	59	66,3%
7	no	62	25,2%	10	17,9%	95	15,3%	12	14,0%
	yes	184	74,8%	46	82,1%	524	84,7%	74	86,0%
8	no	35	14,9%	8	15,1%	53	8,6%	6	7,5%
	yes	200	85,1%	45	84,9%	562	91,4%	74	92,5%
9	no	15	6,5%	6	11,1%	14	2,3%	0	0%
	yes	215	93,5%	48	88,9%	588	97,7%	80	100,0%
12	no	0	0%	0	0%	2	,3%	0	0%
	yes	234	100,0%	52	100,0%	575	99,7%	81	100,0%

Introduction of complementary feeding in five European countries

Sonia A Schiess[1], Veit Grote[2], Silvia Scaglioni[3], Veronica Luque[4], Francoise Martin[5], Anna Stolarczyk[7], Fiammetta Vecchi[3], Joana Hoyos[6], Marta Zaragoza-Jordana M[4], Anna Dobrzanska[7], Berthold Koletzko[1] for the European Childhood Obesity Project *

[1]Div. Metabolic Diseases & Nutritional Medicine, Dr. von Hauner Children's Hospital, Ludwig-Maximilians-University, Munich, Germany [2] Dept. Epidemiology, Inst. of Social Pediatrics and Adolescent Medicine, Ludwig-Maximilians-University, Munich, Germany [3]Dept. of Pediatrics, San Paolo Hospital, Milan, Italy [4]Dept. of Medicine & Surgery Pediatrics Unit, University Rovira i Virgili, Reus, Spain [5]CHC St. Vincent, Rocourt, Belgium [6]Department of Peadiatrics, Université Libre de Bruxelles, Brussels, Belgium [7]Clinic of Pediatrics, Children's Memorial Health Institute, Warsaw, Poland

*Study team:

Belgium (ULB Bruxelles and CHC St Vincent Liège): Carlier C, Goyens P, Langhendries J-P, Van Hees J-N, Xhonneux A; **Germany** (Division of Nutritional Medicine and Metabolism, Dr. von Hauner Children's Hospital, and Division of Pediatric Epidemiology, Institute of Social Pediatrics and Adolescent Medicine, Ludwig-Maximilians-University of Munich): Beyer J, Demmelmair H, Fritsch M, Handel U, Hannibal I, von Kries R, Pawellek I, Verwied-Jorky S; **Italy** (University of Milan): Giovannini M, Agostoni C, Confalonieri F, Marcello, Tedeschi S, Verduci E; **Spain** (Universitat Rovira i Virgili IISPV): Closa Monasterolo R, Escribano Subias J, Méndez Riera G, Ferre N; **Poland** (Children's Memorial Health Institute): Socha J, Gruszfeld D, Socha P, Janas R, Pietraszek E, Kowalik A

Abstract

Background: Little information is available on the practice of introducing complementary feeding across Europe.

Objectives: To describe the times of complementary feeding (CF) introduction in healthy infants in five European countries.

Methods: Infants breast fed for at least three completed months (BF, n=588) and two randomized formula fed infant groups (FF, n=1090) with formula milk of different protein contents were recruited between October 2002 and June 2004. Three-day-weighed food protocols were obtained at the ages of one to nine and again at twelve completed months.

Results: At the age of four completed months, 13% of BF and 43% of FF infants received energy providing liquids (EPL), and 17% of BF and 37% of FF infants received solids, respectively. We found significant differences between countries, with the highest proportion of FF infants consuming EPL in Poland (87%), of BF infants in Spain (26%) and for solid intake in Belgium (FF infants 56%, BF infants 43%). FF infants receiving EPL had a significantly lower formula (at ages 2 to 5 months, $p<0.05$) and solid intake (at ages seven to nine and twelve months, $p<0.05$). Multiple regressions showed the country of residence as strongest factor influencing the time of CF introduction.

Conclusions: EPL and solids were introduced earlier than recommended to a high proportion of infants, particularly among FF infants. Regional differences strongly influenced the time of introduction of CF which should be considered in parental counseling strategies.

Background

In the 1920s infants in the United States consumed sieved vegetable soup by the end of the first year and potatoes with around 18 months of age (1). From 1930 onwards, the age for the introduction of complementary foods (CF) decreased, pediatricians recommended already strained fruit and vegetables at the age of 4 to 6 months. In the 1950s solid introduction was recommended even before 8 weeks of age and there was promotion of feeding strained fruit and vegetables after some days of age. In the early 1970s there was a low initial breastfeeding rate in the United States (<25%), but worldwide tendency of increasing breastfeeding and CF introduction at around six weeks of age. In the 1980s the consumption of fruit juices increased remarkably, as source of nutrients, vitamins and simple carbohydrates but also related to dental caries. Nowadays the introduction of complementary feeding is not recommended before the age of 4 months. The population based recommendation of the World Health Organization (WHO) suggests 6 months of exclusive breastfeeding compared to many industrialized countries where advisory boards stay with the recommendation not to start with CF before 4 to 6 months. Also, EPL are not recommended nor needed in the first months of life. The American Academy of Pediatrics (AAP) sees no nutritional indication to feed infants younger than 6 months with fruit juice and if infants get fruit juices these should be provided from a cup (2).

However, infant feeding practice is suspected to differ considerably from current recommendations. Therefore, we aimed to characterize the practice of introducing EPL and solids to infants in five European countries with similar infant feeding recommendations. Data was collected as part of the prospective European Childhood Obesity Project. We explored whether type of milk feeding, socio-demographic characteristics and the country of residence were associated with the time point of introduction of complementary feeding.

Definition of complementary feeding

The definitions for complementary feeding are not consistent. For the WHO complementary feeding is 'any nutrient-containing foods or liquids other than breast milk' with the aim to emphasize breastfeeding (3). For the European Society for Paediatric Gastroenterology, Hepatology and Nutrition (ESPGHAN) complementary feeding includes 'solid and liquid foods other than breast milk or infant formula and follow-on formula'. In this definition formula milk is not considered as part of the complementary foods to avoid confusion for infants starting with formula milk from the first weeks of life. Others define complementary feeding as anything beside breast milk or formula milk given to the infant or refer to any solids introduced to the infant diet (4-6).

Some considerations

Complementary feeding should be introduced when the nutritional need is not covered anymore through breast milk. For the majority of healthy full term infants, a sufficient volume of breast milk from a well nourished mother should supply the nutrient needs of the infant until about 6 months of age (6;7). However, analysis of Reilly et al. questions if the energy transfer from mother milk is always sufficient for the infant until the age of 6 months (8). Further, micronutrients which can occasionally be deficient before 6 months of age are vitamin D, if very little sunlight reaches the infant's skin or zinc because of the physiological decline in the zinc content of human milk or vitamins like A, B_{12}, and riboflavin (6;7).

In the first months of life, infants should be exclusively breastfed or fed with infant formula and do not require liquids like water, tea, juices, sweetened beverages or other energy providing liquids (EPL) with possible exception in selected conditions such as diarrhea, very high ambient temperatures, high fever or in some special indications occurring in the neonatal period (9).

With the age of 6 months most infants reach a general and neurological stage of development (chewing, swallowing, digestion and excretion) that enables them to be fed by other foods rather than breast milk (10).

Actual recommendations

In 2001, the 54th World Health Assembly recommended the introduction of complementary foods around the 6th month of life, instead between the 4th and 6th month, as previously recommended (11). After the Expert Consultation in 2001 and the WHO-commissioned systematic review by Kramer and Kakuma the global recommendation was modified to six months exclusive breastfeeding with the introduction of complementary feeding thereafter and continued breastfeeding for the first 2 years (12). The advantages include a lower risk of gastrointestinal infection, more rapid maternal weight loss after birth, and delayed return of menstrual periods. No reduced risks of other infections or of allergic diseases have been demonstrated. No adverse effects on growth have been documented with exclusive breastfeeding for 6 months, but a reduced level of iron has been observed in developing-country settings (12). In Europe the recommendations call mostly for 4 to 6 months exclusive breastfeeding followed by a stepwise introduction of the complementary feeding. To avoid the risk that a subgroup of infants could not be covered with some micronutrients by an exclusive breastfeeding of 6 months, an earlier introduction of complementary foods would be beneficial (4). The ESPGHAN considers as desirable goal that infants are exclusively or fully breastfed for 6 months and receive complementary feeding not before 17 weeks and not later than 26 weeks of life (13). The American Academy of Pediatrics (AAP) suggests the introduction of complementary feeding after the age of 4 to 6 months (14). The recommendations in the participating countries of the study agree that complementary feeding should not start before the age of 4 months (15).

Should the recommendations for the introduction of complementary feeding differ between BF infants and FF infants?

For breastfed infants the main micronutrients of concern are iron and zinc, compared to formula fed infants with some greater nutrient density in their standard cows' milk formula (6;7). For this reason Foote mentions the option that breast fed infants should receive foods such as meat or iron fortified foods earlier in the weaning process than formula fed infants, in whom cereals would suffice as the initial solid food (6). Dewey mentions the option to supplement exclusive breastfed infants for 6 months with iron and zinc (16;17). Further, the energy intake and expenditure for formula fed infants has been identified differently in the study of Butte (18) and the growth pattern and weight gain is also different during the first year and later (19-22). The WHO recommendations for complementary feeding take no account of the likely differing nutrient requirements of the exclusively breast fed versus the formula or mixed formula and breast fed infants. Alike, the ESPGHAN prefer to have unanimous recommendations for all infants (13).

Factors influencing an early introduction of complementary foods

Mothers' education and their social environment are known as strong factors influencing the feeding practices of their infants. Depending on the development stage of the society, these factors may favor an earlier or a later introduction of complementary feeding to the infants (4). Infants formula fed, the younger age of the mother and her smoking behavior are more factors associated with an earlier introduction of complementary feeding(23-25).

Possible consequences of an early or late introduction of complementary foods
Energy providing liquids
Feeding infants with EPL may displace breast milk or infant formula intake and thereby, may adversely affect nutrient supply (2;26). Beyond that, regular intake of EPL might prime infants to their sweet taste with a possible increased risk for later development of dental caries or obesity (2;27-29). Further, high and regular intake of fruit juices may exceed the intestine's ability to absorb the carbohydrate and favor risks of malabsorption (26;30). Excess of fruit juice consumption was also associated as contributing factor in some children with nonorganic failure to thrive and decreased stature (26).

Solids
Different studies have associated very early introduction of complementary foods with an increased risk of allergy. The intake of complementary feeding before the age of 4 months seems to increase the risk of allergies as well as if introduced after 7 months (14;31-36). Further, a late introduction of complementary foods could be disadvantageous, because infant growth stops or slows down, the risk of malnutrition and micronutrient deficiency increases (10) and it may trigger to unwanted feeding behavior later on (37). Northstone et al. found that infants with a late introduction of lumpy solids were associated with increased difficulties in feeding in older ages (5).

Kleinman in his analysis did not find clear associations between the age of introduction of complementary foods and cancer, later obesity, hypertension, coronary vascular disease or osteoporosis (38).

Study design
Data were collected as part of the European Childhood Obesity Project, a double-blind, randomized controlled trial with one group of breastfed (BF) infants and two groups of formula fed (FF) infants randomized to formula with different protein levels as a possible risk factor for later obesity. The methodology of the study has been previously reported (39;40). In short, eligible participants were apparently healthy, singletons, term infants who were born between 1 October 2002 and 30 June 2004 and followed in 11 study centers in five European countries (Belgium, Germany, Italy, Poland and Spain). Exclusion criteria were mothers with hormonal or metabolic diseases or illicit addiction during pregnancy (40). The first medical visit included infant anthropometry measurements as well as collection of socioeconomic data, medical histories of parents and infants. During the

following months, parents and infants were followed at regular intervals in the study centers, as well as by mailed questionnaires on feeding behaviors. For dietary data collection a 3-day weighed food protocol at the age of 1 to 9 and again 12 completed months was chosen (41). Trained dieticians in all study centers entered the data of the food protocols from their centre using a special software developed for this study. Complementary foods (3281 food items) consumed during the first year of life by the infants in the five countries were classified based on their major ingredients and categorized into subgroups. For our analysis solids included food items such as beef, cereals or bread, egg, fat, fish, fruit, meat, milk or milk products, nuts or seeds, potatoes, poultry, pulses, sausages, soy or soy products, sweets or infant sweets and vegetables. Energy providing liquids (EPL) were defined as sugared instant tea, fruit juices (100% fruit juice, fruit drinks) and vegetable juices provided as drinks (but not as one ingredient of a composed dish), and other sugared beverages (soft drinks, sugared water without or with flavors).

Mothers were grouped in four categories based on age at birth (I=≤25, II=>25 to 30, III= >30 to 35 and IV=>35 years) and the maternal educational levels were categorized in 3 groups (*low* =pre-preliminary to lower secondary, *middle* = upper secondary and post-secondary non-tertiary and *high* = first and second stage of tertiary education).

For data analysis Stata 9.2, SPSS 16.0 and Excel 2000 were used. Chi square and multiple logistic regression analysis were used to adjust differences in the time points of solid or EPL introduction at each month by confounders. The study protocol was reviewed and accepted by the ethic committees at all study centers.

Discussion

The data analysis shows that EPL and solids were given to a very high proportion of European infants already during the first months of life (15;41) (**Figure 1**). At the age of four months, 13% of BF infants and 43% of FF infants had already received EPL, and 17% of BF infants and 37 % of FF infants consumed solids, even though such an early introduction is not supported at all by current recommendations (11;13). Also other studies reported discordance between infant feeding recommendations and practice. In the Euro-Growth Study, 50%, 67%, and 95% of infants were fed some solid foods at the ages of three, four, and five months, respectively (42). Giovannini et al. found around 6% of infants with solid introduction before the age of 3 months and 34% at the age of 4 months (43). Also in the United Kingdom many infants received complementary food far earlier than suggested (6;44).

There is no nutritional benefit of feeding EPL or fruit juices to infants during the first months of life, but there is a possible risk of displacing nutrient intakes from breast milk or infant formula as previously proposed (45-47). Our data analyses confirm a lower formula milk intake (kcal/d) in FF infants who consumed EPL during the first months of life (41) (**Figure 2**). Furthermore, infants who consumed EPL had a lower solids intake (kcal/d) during the second half of the first year (**Figure 3**). Thus, the provision of EPL can displace the intake of other foods and the supply of relevant nutrients with these foods. The use of EPL is also associated with early introduction of solids: infants who received EPL had significantly higher energy intakes from solids at the ages of 4 and 5 months as compared to infants who did not receive EPL. An early introduction of solids, prior to the age of 3 and 4 completed months, was associated with an increased risk of eczema, celiac disease, and allergy (35;36;48-50).

Introduction of complementary feeding is recommended at the same age for both FF and BF infants, but FF infants received both EPL and solids earlier than BF infants, which is consistent with previous findings (15;44;51-54) (**Figure 1**). In our study, FF infants were five times more likely to receive EPL by the age of four months than BF infants. Higher parental socioeconomic status and educational level, as well as exclusive breastfeeding during the first months of life, were associated with later complementary feeding introduction.

Our study involved five European countries with different cultural traditions and food patterns. Even though guidelines for the introduction of complementary foods are similar in these countries, there are significant differences in infant feeding practice between the countries, both in FF and BF infants (15) (**Table 1**). During the first year of life, we found the highest percentages of BF infants with consumption of EPL in Poland and Spain and of FF infants in Poland (41). At the age of four months, we found the highest percentages of BF infants (43%) and FF infants (56%) with introduction of solids in Belgium (15). This earlier introduction, compared to other countries, is not due to different recommendations in Poland or Belgium and remains unexplained.

The strongest risk factors for early introduction of solids in FF infants at the age of 3 completed months were country of residence and young maternal age, and at 4 months the country of residence, low maternal education and maternal smoking. In BF infants the country of residence and lower maternal education level were associated with introduction of solids at the age of 4 completed months. These findings were consistent with other studies also finding earlier introduction of complementary feeding in children of lower parental educational level (55), lower socioeconomic status (24), maternal smoking(23;25) and younger maternal age (56).

While we found no differences in the timing of introducing complementary foods between infants randomized to the two types of intervention formulas with different protein and fat contents, there were significant differences between countries in the timing of introducing complementary foods (**Table 1**). This observation suggests far stronger effects of regional and cultural traditions, as well as social and parental factors on the time of introducing complementary foods than of dietary macronutrient composition.

In conclusion, complementary foods as EPL or solids are provided much earlier to many infants, particularly FF infants, than currently recommended. There are marked differences between the five European countries of our study in the timing of introducing EPL and solids. The provision of EPL is associated with a lower energy intake from infant formula, earlier introduction of solids, and less energy intake from solids during the second half of the first year of life. There is room for improvement in infant feeding practices, particularly in risk groups including infants fed formula and infants of mothers with lower level of education, younger age or smoking behavior.

Acknowledgements

We are extremely grateful to the parents and their infants who participated in this study and to the physicians, midwives and nurses for their helpful support in recruiting mothers during pregnancy or after giving birth. We want to thank the CHOP team for their effort and dedication, the dieticians for the patience to complete the nutritional data and Fabio Confalionieri for his support of the NutrCalc software.

Authors' contributions:

SSch: enrolment of subjects, acquisition and introduction of data, data analysis and interpretation, manuscript writing. VG: data management and data analysis, contribute to manuscript writing. SSc: participated in study design and conduct of study, contribute to manuscript writing. VL, FM, AS, FV: enrolment of subjects, conduct of study, acquisition and introduction of data, contribute to manuscript writing. BK: principal investigator and guarantor of the study, contribution to manuscript writing. All authors read and approved the final version of the article.

Conflict of interest:

None of the authors has declared a conflict of interest.

Funding

The European Childhood Obesity Programme is being carried out with financial support of the European Community, under the 5th Framework Programme for Research, Technology & Demonstration „Quality of Life and Management of Living Resources", Key Action 1 (Food, Nutrition & Health), contract number QLK1-CT2002-389.

The study was carried out with financial support of the European Community, under the 5th Framework Programme for Research, Technology & Demonstration „Quality of Life and Management of Living Resources", Key Action 1 (Food, Nutrition & Health), contract number QLK1-CT2002-389. Berthold Koletzko is the recipient of a Freedom to Discover Award of the Bristol Myers Squibb Foundation, New York, NY, USA.

The presented data are part of the PhD Thesis in Human Biology submitted by Sonia A. Schiess to the Medical Faculty, Ludwig-Maximilian-University of Munich.

Reference List

1. Fomon SJ. Infant Feeding in the 20th Century: Formula and Beikost. J Nutr 2001;131:409S-420.
2. Committee on Nutrition. The Use and Misuse of Fruit Juice in Pediatrics. Pediatrics 2001;107:1210-3.
3. WHO. Complementary feeding of young children in developing countries: A review of current scientific knowledge. WHO 1998;WHO/NUT/98.1.
4. Lanigan JA, Bishop JA, Kimber AC, Morgan J. Review: Systemic review concerning the age of introduction of complementary foods to the healthy full-term infant. European Journal of Clinical Nutrition 2001;55:309-20.
5. Northstone K, Emmett P, Nethersole F. The effect of age of introduction to lumpy solids on foods eaten and reported feeding difficulties at 6 and 15 months. Journal of Human Nutrition and Dietetics 2001;14:43-54.
6. Foote KD, Marriott LD. Weaning of infants. Arch Dis Child 2003;88:488-92.
7. Dewey KG. Nutrition, growth and complementary feeding of the breastfed infant. In: Hale TW, Hartmann P, eds. Human lactation. Amarillo, TX: Hale Publishing, 2007:415-23.
8. Reilly JJ, Wells JCK. Duration of exclusive breast-feeding: introduction of complementary feeding may be necessary before 6 months of age. British Journal of Nutrition 2005;94:869-72.
9. Kersting M. Ernährung des gesunden Säuglings. Monatsschrift Kinderheilkunde 2001;149:4-10.
10. Monte CMG, Giugliani ERJ. Recommendations for the complementary feeding of the breastfed child. J Pediatr (Rio J) 2004;80 (5Suppl):S131-S141.
11. WHO 54th World Health Assembly. Infant and young child nutrition. WHA54.2.
12. Kramer MS, Kakuma R. Optimal duration of exclusive breastfeeding. Cochrane Database Syst Rev 2002;Issue 1. Art.No.: CD003517. DOI:10.1002/14651858:CD003517.
13. ESPGHAN Committee of Nutrition: Agostoni C, Decsi T, Fewtrell M et al. Complementary feeding: a commentary by the ESPGHAN Committee on Nutrition. J Pediatr Gastroenterol Nutr 2008;46:99-110.

14. Greer FR, Sicherer SH, Burks AW, and the Committee on Nutrition and Section on Allergy and Immunology. Effects of Early Nutritional Interventions on the Development of Atopic Disease in Infants and Children: The Role of Maternal Dietary Restriction, Breastfeeding, Timing of Introduction of Complementary Foods, and Hydrolyzed Formulas. Pediatrics 2008;121:183-91.
15. Schiess S, Grote V, Scaglioni S et al. Introduction of complementary feeding in five European countries. J Pediatr Gastroenterol Nutr 2010;50(1):92-8.
16. Dewey KG. What is the optimal age for introduction of complementary foods ? Nestle Nutr Workshop Ser Pediatr Program 2006;58:161-75.
17. PAHO and WHO. Guiding principles for feeding non-breastfed children 6-24 months of age. WHO. WHO , 1-42. Ref Type: Report.
18. Butte NF, Wong WW, Ferlic L, Smith EO, Klein PD, Garza C. Energy expenditure and deposition of breast-fed and formula-fed infants during early infancy [published erratum appeared in Pediatr Res 1991 May;29(5):454]. Pediatr Res 1990;28:631-40.
19. Heinig MJ, Nommsen LA, Peerson JM, Lonnerdal B, Dewey KG. Energy and protein intakes of breast-fed and formula-fed infants during the first year of life and their association with growth velocity: the DARLING Study. Am J Clin Nutr 1993;58:152-61.
20. Dewey KG. Nutrition, growth, and complementary feeding of the breastfed infant. Pediatr Clin North Am 2001;48 (1):87-104.
21. Hediger ML, Overpeck MD, Ruan WJ, Troendle JF. Early infant feeding and growth status of US-born infants and children aged 4-71 mo: analyses from the third National Health and Nutrition Examination Survey, 1988-1994. Am J Clin Nutr 2000;72:159-67.
22. Butte NF, Wong WW, Hopkinson JM, Smith EO, Ellis KJ. Infant Feeding Mode Affects Early Growth and Body Composition. Pediatrics 2000;106:1355-66.
23. Ford RP, Schluter PJ, Mitchell EA. Factors associated with the age of introduction of solids into the diet of new Zealand infants. New Zealand Cot Death Study Group. J Paediatr Child Health 1995;31(5):469-72.
24. Alder EM, Williams FL, Anderson AS, Forsyth S, Florey C, van der Velde P. What influence the timing of the introduction of solid food to infants ? British Journal of Nutrition 2004;92(3):527-31.
25. Ratner PA, Johnson JL, Bottorff JL. Smoking Relapse and Early Weaning Among Postpartum Women: Is There an Association? Birth 1999;26:76-82.

26. Dennison BA. Fruit juice consumption by infants and children: a review. J Am Coll Nutr 1996;15(5):4S-11S.
27. Ludwig DS, Peterson KE, Gortmaker SL. Relation between consumption of sugar-sweetened drinks and childhood obesity: a prospective, observational analysis. The Lancet 2001;357:505-8.
28. Malik VS, Schulze MB, Hu FB. Intake of sugar-sweetened beverages and weight gain: a systematic review. Am J Clin Nutr 2006;84:274-88.
29. Vartanian LR, Schwartz MB, Brownell KD. Effects of soft drink consumption on nutrition and health: a systematic review and meta-analysis. Am J Public Health 2007;97(4):667-75.
30. Smith MM, Davis M, Chasalow FI, Lifshitz F. Carbohydrate Absorption From Fruit Juice in Young Children. Pediatrics 1995;95:340-4.
31. Wilson AC, Forsyth JS, Greene SA, Irvine L, Hau C, Howie PW. Relation of infant diet to childhood health: seven year follow up of cohort of children in Dundee infant feeding study. BMJ 1998;316:21-5.
32. Oddy WH, Holt PG, Sly PD et al. Association between breast feeding and asthma in 6 year old children: findings of a prospective birth cohort study. BMJ 1999;319:815-9.
33. Zutavern A, Brockow I, Schaaf B et al. Timing of Solid Food Introduction in Relation to Atopic Dermatitis and Atopic Sensitization: Results From a Prospective Birth Cohort Study. Pediatrics 2006;117:401-11.
34. Zutavern A, Brockow I, Schaaf B et al. Timing of solid food introduction in relation to eczema, asthma, allergic rhinitis, and food and inhalant sensitization at the age of 6 years: results from the prospective birth cohort study LISA. Pediatrics 2008;121:e44-e52.
35. Ziegler A-G, Schmid S, Huber D, Hummel M, Bonifacio E. Early Infant Feeding and Risk of Developing Type 1 Diabetes-Associated Autoantibodies. JAMA 2003;290:1721-8.
36. Norris JM, Barriga K, Klingensmith G et al. Timing of Initial Cereal Exposure in Infancy and Risk of Islet Autoimmunity. JAMA 2003;290:1713-20.
37. Paine P, Spergiorin C. Prolonged breast feeding related to later solid food acceptance. Child: Care, Health and Development 1983;9:321-6.
38. Kleinmann RE. Complementary feeding and later health. Pediatrics 2000;106(5):1287S.

39. Koletzko B, von Kries R, Monasterolo RC et al. Can infant feeding choices modulate later obesity risk? Am J Clin Nutr 2009;89(5):S1502-S1508.
40. Koletzko B, von Kries R, Monasterolo RC et al. Lower protein in infant formula is associated with lower weight up to age 2 y: a randomized clinical trial. Am J Clin Nutr 2009;89:1-10.
41. Schiess SA, Grote V, Scaglioni S et al. Intake of energy providing liquids during the first year of life in five European countries. Clinical Nutrition 2010;in press.
42. Freeman V, Van´t Hof M, Haschke F. Patterns of milk and food intake in infants from birth to age 36 months: the Euro-Growth Study. J Pediatr Gastroenterol Nutr 2000;31 Suppl 1:S76-S85.
43. Giovannini M, Riva E, Banderali G et al. Feeding practices of infants through the first year of life in Italy. Acta Paediatr 2004;93:492-7.
44. Wright CM, Parkinson KN, Drewett RF. Why are babies weaned early? Data from a prospective population based cohort study. Arch Dis Child 2004;89:813-6.
45. Marshall TLS, Broffitt B, Eichenberger-Gilmore J, Stumbo J. Beverage consumption and infant nutrition - Benefits of milk vs. juice. Nutrition Research Newsletter 2003.
46. Saalfield S, Jackson-Allen P. Biopsychosocial consequences of sweetened drink consumption in children 0-6 years of age. Pediatric Nursing 2006;32(5):460-71.
47. Gibson SA. Non-milk extrinsic sugars in the diets of pre-school children: association with intakes of micronutrients, energy, fat and NSP. British Journal of Nutrition 1997;78:367-78.
48. Fergusson DM, Horwood LJ, Shannon FT. Early Solid Feeding and Recurrent Childhood Eczema: A 10-Year Longitudinal Study. Pediatrics 1990;86:541-6.
49. Morgan J, Williams P, Norris F, Williams C, Larkin M, Hampton S. Eczema and early solid feeding in preterm infants. Arch Dis Child 2004;89:309-14.
50. Norris JM, Barriga K, Hoffenberg EJ et al. Risk of Celiac Disease Autoimmunity and Timing of Gluten Introduction in the Diet of Infants at Increased Risk of Disease. JAMA 2005;293:2343-51.
51. Parada C, Carvalhaes MABL.Jamas MT. Complementary feeding practices to children during their first year of life. Rev Latino Am Enfermagem 2007;15(2):282-9.
52. Emmett, P., North, K., Noble, S., and ALSPAC Study Team. Types of drinks consumed by infants at 4 and 8 months of age: a descriptive study. Public Health Nutrition 3(2), 211-217.

53. van den Boom.S.A.M., Kimber AC, Morgan JB. Weaning practices in children up to 19 months of age in Madrid. Acta Paediatr 1995;84:853-8.
54. Lande.B., Andersen.L.F., Baerug A et al. Infant feeding practices and associated factors in the first six months of life: The Norwegian Infant Nutrition Survey. Acta Paediatr 2003;92:152-61.
55. Hendricks K, Briefel R, Novak T, Ziegler P. Maternal and Child Characteristics Associated with Infant and Toddler Feeding Practices. Journal of the American Dietetic Association 2006;106:135-48.
56. Savage SA, Reilly JJ, Edwards CA, Durnin JVGA. Weaning practice in the Glasgow longitudinal infant growth study. Arch Dis Child 1998;79:153-6.

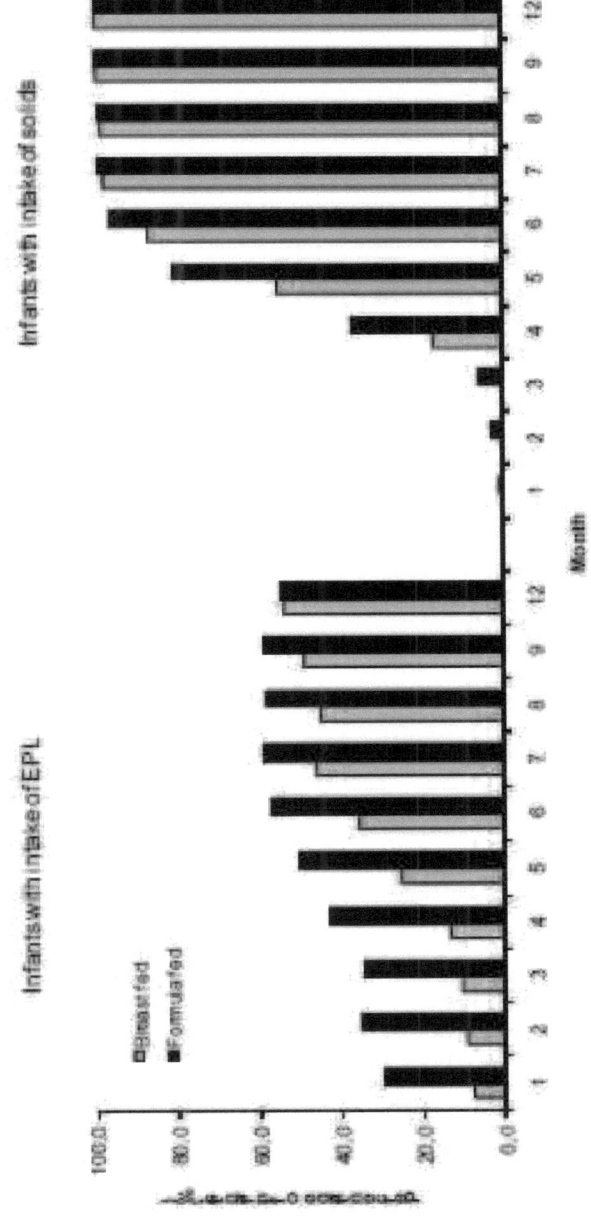

Figure 1: Percentages of breast fed infants and formula fed infants with intake of energy providing liquids (EPL) and solids during the first year of life

Figure 2: The median energy intake (kcal/d) from formula milk in formula fed infants with and without consumption of energy providing liquid (EPL), at the ages of 1 to 9 and 12 completed months

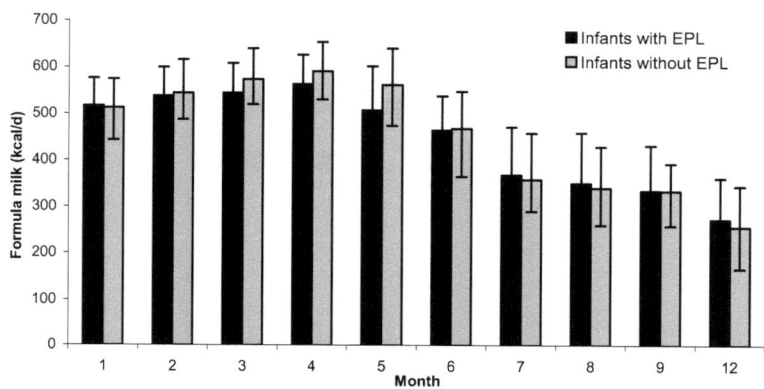

Kruskall-Wallis: 2nd to 5th month p<0.05

Figure 3: The median energy intake (kcal/d) from solids in formula fed infants with and without consumption of energy providing liquid (EPL), at the ages of 1 to 9 and 12 completed months

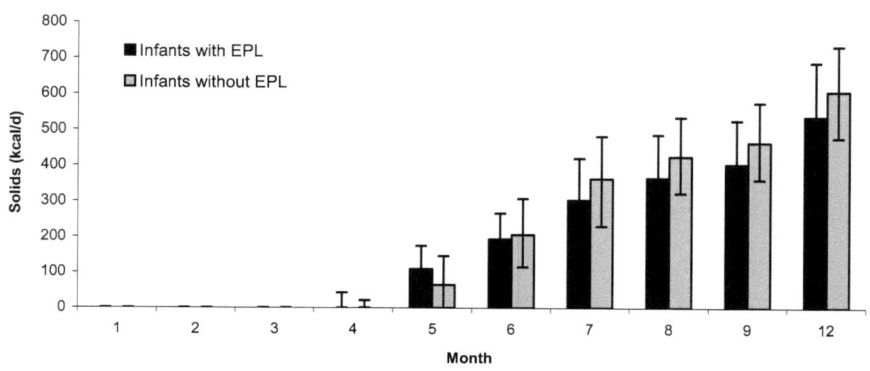

Kruskall-Wallis: 4th to 5th month p<0.01; 7th to 9th and 12th month p<0.001

Table 1: Percentages of breast fed infants and formula fed infants with energy providing liquids and solid introduction, divided by country at the ages 1 to 7 completed months

EPL	Age (completed months)						
BF infants	1	2^1	3^1	4^1	5^1	6^1	7^1
Germany	4	4	2	3	12	25	38
Belgium	0	3	4	14	24	31	40
Italy	8	15	14	9	18	28	34
Poland	14	16	21	18	34	52	73
Spain	10	3	7	26	45	53	63
FF infants	1^2	2^2	3^2	4^2	5^2	6^2	7^2
Germany	34	37	35	44	47	60	61
Belgium	1	3	4	12	26	38	46
Italy	25	28	27	33	33	37	38
Poland	88	79	81	87	93	94	94
Spain	27	25	22	35	48	56	61

Solids							
BF infants	1	2	3	4^2	5^2	6^2	7
Germany	0	1	0	5	25	69	93
Belgium	0	0	0	43	85	96	100
Italy	0	1	1	15	59	93	99
Poland	0	0	0	7	36	84	98
Spain	3	0	1	26	70	89	98
FF infants	1^1	2^1	3^1	4^1	5^1	6^1	7^1
Germany	0	4	5	31	68	91	97
Belgium	5	10	16	56	75	94	100
Italy	0	1	2	31	81	98	100
Poland	3	3	3	39	94	97	100
Spain	1	2	8	38	80	97	100

[1] Chi square $p \leq 0.01$, [2] Chi square $p \leq 0.001$

Zusammenfassung

Im EU Childhood Obesity Projekt (http://www.metabolic-programming.org), einer doppelt blind randomisierten Interventionsstudie mit über 1000 gesunden, reifgeborenen Säuglingen aus fünf europäischen Ländern (Belgien, Deutschland, Italien, Polen und Spanien), wird der Zusammenhang zwischen der Eiweißzufuhr im Säuglingsalter und der Entwicklung von Wachstum und Gewicht bei Kindern nach der Geburt bis zum Alter von 8.5 Jahren untersucht. Das Studienkollektiv besteht aus einer Kontrollgruppe gestillter Säuglinge (n=588) und zwei randomisierten Interventionsgruppen nicht gestillter Säuglinge (n=1090), die bis zur achten Lebenswoche auf eine der Studien-Säuglingsanfangsnahrungen mit unterschiedlichem Eiweißgehalt umgestellten wurden. Innerhalb des EU Childhood Obestiy Projektes wurde der Frage nachgegangen, ob der unterschiedliche Eiweißgehalt in den Säuglingsanfangsnahrungen Einfluss auf den zeitlichen Beginn der Beikosteinführung hat.

Anhand von monatlichen 3-Tage Wiegeprotokolle wurde der Zeitpunkt der Beikosteinführung bei gestillten Säuglingen im Vergleich zu nicht gestillten Säuglingen ermittelt. So auch der Zeitpunkt der Einführung von energiehaltigen Getränken und potentiell allergenen Nahrungsmitteln.

Die Resultate zeigen, dass gestillte und nicht gestillte Säuglinge in einem hohen Prozentsatz Beikost einschließlich potentiell allergenen Nahrungsmittel wie auch energiehaltige Getränke vor dem empfohlenem Alter von vier Monaten erhielten. Trotz gleicher Empfehlungen, bekamen nicht gestillte Säuglinge zu einem signifikant früheren Zeitpunkt und zu signifikant höheren Anteilen feste Beikost, energiehaltige Getränke wie auch potentiell allergene Nahrungsmittel im Vergleich zu gestillten Säuglingen. Im Alter von vier Monaten verzehrten 17% der gestillten Säuglinge feste Beikost und 13% energiehaltige Getränke. Im gleichem Alter bekamen 37% der Säuglinge mit Säuglingsanfangsnahrung feste Beikost und 43% energiehaltige Getränke. Die Zufuhr von energiehaltigen Getränken wirkte sich signifikant auf eine geringere Aufnahme von Säuglingsanfangsnahrung im Alter von zwei, drei, vier und fünf Monaten ($p<0.05$), sowie auch eine signifikant geringere Beikostzufuhr im Alter von sieben, acht, neun und zwölf Monaten aus ($p<0.05$). Im Alter von 4 Monaten verzehrten 6% der gestillten und 13% der nicht gestillten Säuglinge potentiell allergene Nahrungsmittel. Mütter mit Allergien verabreichten ihren Säuglingen in einem früheren Alter potentiell allergene Nahrungsmittel als Mütter ohne Allergien. Weiterhin fanden sich trotz ähnlicher Empfehlungen signifikante Unterschiede zwischen den Ländern im Bezug auf die zeitliche Einführung von Beikost, ob als feste Nahrungsmittel oder als energiehaltige Getränke, bei den gestillten sowie nicht gestillten Säuglingen. Die unterschiedliche Nährstoffzusammensetzung der Studien-Säuglingsanfangsnahrung hatte keinen Einfluss auf das Alter der Beikosteinführung. Der Ausbildungsgrad der Mutter, das Alter der Mutter wie auch ihre Rauchgewohnheiten hatten einen signifikanten Einfluss auf den Zeitpunkt der Beikosteinführung. Eine gute Information und Aufklärung an die Eltern, speziell von Säuglingen, die Säuglingsanfangsnahrung erhalten, über die zeitlich korrekte Einführung der Beikost, in fester und flüssiger Form wäre sehr wünschenswert.

Summary

The European Childhood Obesity Project (http://www.metabolic-programming.org), a double blind randomized intervention trial with over 1000 healthy, term infants from five European countries (Belgium, Germany, Italy, Poland and Spain) will analyse the relation of the infant protein supply and the growth and weight development after birth up to the age of 8.5 years. The study population included one reference group of infants fully breastfed for at least three months (n=588) and two groups of formula fed infants (n=1090) randomized to the higher or lower protein formula, latest at the age of eight weeks. As part of the prospective EU Childhood Obesity Project we aimed at analyzing if the different protein content of the formula milk had some influence of the time point of introduction of complementary feeding. With the dietary data collected by the three-day-weighed food records the time point of introduction of complementary feeding of breast fed (BF) and formula fed (FF) infants were analysed as well as for the time point of introduction of energy providing liquids and potential allergenic foods.

The results showed a high percentage of breast fed and formula fed infants with intake of solids, energy providing liquids and potential allergenic foods before the recommended age of four completed months of life. Despite similar recommendations, there was a significant earlier introduction and a significant higher percentage of formula fed infants consuming solids, energy providing liquids and potential allergenic foods compared to breast fed infants. At the age of four completed months, already 37% of FF infants and 17% of BF infants consumed solids and 43% of FF infants and 13% of BF infants consumed energy providing liquids. Formula fed infants with energy providing liquid intake had a significant lower intake of formula milk at the age of two to five months ($p<0.05$) and solid intake at the age of seven to nine and twelve months ($p<0.05$). Some 6% of BF infants and 13% of FF infants consumed some potential allergenic food at the age of four completed months. Mothers with history of allergy introduced earlier potential allergenic foods to their infants than mothers without history of allergy.

Although there are similar national recommendations, we found significant differences in the time point of introduction of solids and energy providing liquid between the countries in breast fed and formula fed infants. There was no association between the protein contents of study formula and the time point of introduction of complementary feeding. The educational level of the mother, the maternal age and her smoking habits were significantly related to the time point of introduction of complementary feeding. Improved information and education to the parents, especially in formula fed infants, on the correct timing for the introduction of complementary foods, as solids and as beverage would be desirable.

Danksagung

Mein herzlichster Dank an Prof. Dr. Berthold Koletzko für seine Einladung an mich, als Doktorandin am EU Childhood Projekt teilzunehmen. In dieser Zeit habe ich seine Ratschläge, sein Vertrauen wie auch seine freundliche und geduldige Betreuung besonders geschätzt. Durch diese Mitarbeit habe ich viel über selbstständiges, wissenschaftliches Arbeiten im internationalen Rahmen gelernt, wie auch über Datenanalyse und die Daten und Texte kritisch zu beurteilen.

Ein großen Dank an Dr. Hans Demmelmair für seine praktische Hilfen und analytisches Mitdenken, ebenso für seine Geduld und große Hilfsbereitschaft.

Sehr froh und dankbar war ich über die ausdauernde Hilfe von Dr. Veit Grote bei der Zusammensetzung der Datensätze und seiner Unterstützung in der Auswertung der Datenbank.

Den interessanten und wertvollen Austausch mit meinen Studienkollegen/in möchte ich nicht missen und danke allen besonders für ihre Hilfe und ihren Einsatz bei der Zusammenstellung der Beikostliste.

Ganz besonders möchte ich mich bei unseren Studienteilnehmern, Säuglingen und Eltern, für ihre Zeit und Ihren Einsatz bedanken, bei ihren regelmäßigen Besuchen in die Studienzentren wie auch durch das Ausfüllen der vielen Fragebögen und Ernährungsprotokolle. Ohne ihren Einsatz wäre diese Studie gar nicht möglich gewesen.

Sehr geschätzt habe ich den Austausch mit meinen Arbeitskollegen/in, es war eine wertvolle Zeit und danke auch allen für ihre vielseitige Hilfsbereitschaft.

Zum Schluss auch noch ein großes Dankeschön an meine Familie und Freunden, für all ihr Verständnis und ihre Unterstützung während dieser Jahre.

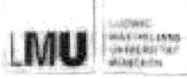 

Kumulative Dissertation

Bestätigung gem. § 4a Abs. 3 und 5 Promotionsordnung

Bon a.A. Schiess
Doktorand/in

Einführung von Beikost in 5 europäischen Ländern
Titel der Dissertation

Hiermit bestätige ich, dass keiner der zur Promotion eingereichten Fachartikel Gegenstand einer anderen laufenden oder abgeschlossenen Dissertation ist.

Unterschrift Doktorand/in

Folgende Ko-Autoren bestätigen hiermit ihr Einverständnis

- Ihren Arbeitsanteil (Inhalt und Umfang) an den eingereichten Veröffentlichungen.
- Ihr Einverständnis zur Einreichung der Publikationen sowie,
- dass der jeweilige eingereichte Fachartikel nicht Gegenstand einer anderen laufenden oder abgeschlossenen Dissertation ist.

Name Ko-Autor	Arbeitsanteil (Inhalt und Umfang)	Unterschrift Ko-Autor
1. Ivan Gross	Data management and data analysis, contribute to manuscript writing	
2. Silvia Scaglioni	participated in study design and conduct of study, contribute to manuscript writing	
3. Veronica Luque	enrolment of subjects, conduct of study, acquisition and introduction of data, contribute to manuscript writing, SOPs	
4. Françoise Martin	enrolment of subjects, conduct of study, acquisition and introduction of data, contribute to manuscript writing	
5. Anna Stolarczyk	enrolment of subjects, conduct of study, acquisition and introduction of data, contribute to manuscript writing	

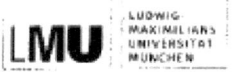 Medizinische Fakultät

Kumulative Dissertation

Bestätigung gem. § 4a Abs. 3 und 5 Promotionsordnung

Sonia A. Schiess
Doktorand

Einführung von Beikost in fünf europäischen Ländern
Titel der Dissertation

Hiermit bestätige ich, dass keiner der zur Promotion eingereichten Fachartikel Gegenstand einer anderen (laufenden oder abgeschlossenen) Dissertation ist.

Unterschrift Doktorand

Folgende **Ko-Autoren** bestätigen mit ihrer Unterschrift

- ihren Arbeitsanteil (Inhalt und Umfang) an den eingereichten Veröffentlichungen,
- ihr Einverständnis zur Einreichung der Publikationen sowie,
- dass der jeweilige eingereichte Fachartikel nicht Gegenstand einer anderen (laufenden oder abgeschlossenen) Dissertation ist.

Name Ko-Autor	Arbeitsanteil (Inhalt und Umfang)	Unterschrift Ko-Autor
1. Veit Grote	data management and data analysis, contribute to manuscript writing	
2. Silvia Scaglioni	participated in study design and conduct of study, contribute to manuscript writing.	
3. Veronica Luque	enrolment of subjects, conduct of study, acquisition and introduction of data, contribute to manuscript writing, SOPS	
4. Francoise Martin	enrolment of subjects, conduct of study, acquisition and introduction of data, contribute to manuscript writing.	
5. Anna Stolarczyk	enrolment of subjects, conduct of study, acquisition and introduction of data, contribute to manuscript writing.	

weitere Autoren bitte auf ein gesondertes Blatt

Kumulative Dissertation - Bestätigung   Stand_27.04.2009

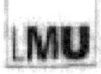 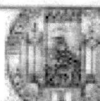

Kumulative Dissertation

Bestätigung gem. § 4a Abs. 3 und 8 Promotionsordnung

Sonja A. Schloss
Doktorand

Einführung von Biologics in fünf europäischen Ländern
Titel der Dissertation

Hiermit bestätige ich, dass keiner der zur Promotion eingereichten Facharbeit Gegenstand einer anderen laufenden oder abgeschlossenen Dissertation ist.

Unterschrift Doktorand

Nachgende Ko-Autoren bestätigen mit ihrer Unterschrift:
- Ihren Arbeitsanteil (Inhalt und Umfang) an den eingereichten Veröffentlichungen.
- Ihr Einverständnis zur Einreichung der Publikationen sowie
- dass der jeweilige eingereichte Facharbeit nicht Gegenstand einer anderen laufenden oder abgeschlossenen Dissertation ist.

Name Ko-Autor	Arbeitsanteil (Inhalt und Umfang)	Unterschrift Ko-Autor
1. Wolf Grote	data management and data analysis, contribute to manuscript writing	
2. Silvia Scaglioni	participated in study design and conduct of study, contribute to manuscript writing	
3. Veronica Luque	enrolment of subjects, conduct of study, acquisition and introduction of data, contribute to manuscript writing, SOPs	
4. Francoise Martin	enrolment of subjects, conduct of study, acquisition and introduction of data, contribute to manuscript writing	Martin
5. Anna Stolarczyk	enrolment of subjects, conduct of study, acquisition and introduction of data, contribute to manuscript writing	

Kumulative Dissertation – Bestätigung

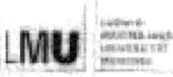

Kumulative Dissertation

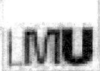 

Kumulative Dissertation

Bestätigung gem. § 4a Abs. 3 und 5 Promotionsordnung

Nasan + Schaas

Einreichung von Bewaat in fünf aamazilischen Ländern

Hiermit bestätige ich, dass keiner der zur Promotion eingereichten Fachartikel Gegenstand einer anderen Bachelor- oder Masterarbeit oder Dissertation ist.

Folgende Ko-Autoren bestätigen mit ihrer Unterschrift:

- ihren Arbeitsanteil, Inhalt und Umfang an der eingereichten Veröffentlichungen,
- ihr Einverständnis zur Einreichung der Publikationen sowie,
- dass der jeweilige eingereichte Fachartikel nicht Gegenstand einer anderen Bachelor- oder Masterarbeit oder Dissertation ist.

Name Ko-Autor	Arbeitsanteil Inhalt und Umfang	Unterschrift Ko-Autor
1. Pigmonella Vaschi	conception of subjects, conduct of study, supervision and introduction of data, contribute to manuscript writing	
2. Berthold Koessko	promoter, investigator and guarantor of the study, designed study protocol, contributed to writing of the manuscript	
3.		
4.		
5.		

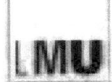 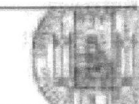

Kumulative Dissertation

Bestätigung gem. §4a Abs. 3 und 5 Promotionsordnung

Sabine A. Schiess

Doktorand/in

Einführung von Beikost in fünf europäischen Ländern

Titel der Dissertation

Hiermit bestätige ich, dass keiner der zur Promotion eingereichten Fachartikel Gegenstand einer anderen laufenden oder abgeschlossenen Dissertation ist.

_____
(Unterschrift Doktorand)

Folgende Ko-Autoren bestätigen mit ihrer Unterschrift

- ihren Arbeitsanteil (Inhalt und Umfang) an den eingereichten Veröffentlichungen,
- ihr Einverständnis zur Einreichung der Publikationen sowie,
- dass der jeweilige eingereichte Fachartikel nicht Gegenstand einer anderen laufenden oder abgeschlossenen Dissertation ist.

Name Ko-Autor	Arbeitsanteil (Inhalt und Umfang)	Unterschrift Ko-Autor
1. Fiammetta Vecchi	enrolment of subjects, conduct of study, acquisition and interpretation of data, contribute to manuscript writing	
2. Berthold Koletzko	principal investigator and guarantor of the study, designed study protocol, contributed to writing of the manuscript	
3.		
4.		
5.		

weiteren Autoren bitte auf ein gesondertes Blatt

Kumulative Dissertation – Bestätigung

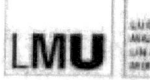 Medizinische Fakultät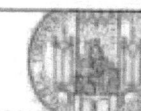

Kumulative Dissertation

Bestätigung gem. § 4a Abs. 3 und 5 Promotionsordnung

Sonia A. Schiess
Doktorand

Einführung von Beikost in fünf europäischen Ländern
Titel der Dissertation

Hiermit bestätige ich, dass keiner der zur Promotion eingereichten Fachartikel Gegenstand einer anderen laufenden oder abgeschlossenen Dissertation ist.

Unterschrift Doktorand

Folgende **Ko-Autoren** bestätigen mit ihrer Unterschrift:

- ihren Arbeitsanteil (Inhalt und Umfang) an den eingereichten Veröffentlichungen,
- ihr Einverständnis zur Einreichung der Publikationen sowie,
- dass der jeweilige eingereichte Fachartikel nicht Gegenstand einer anderen laufenden oder abgeschlossenen Dissertation ist.

Name Ko-Autor	Arbeitsanteil (Inhalt und Umfang)	Unterschrift Ko-Autor
1. Fiammetta Vecchi	enrolment of subjects, conduct of study, acquisition and introduction of data, contribute to manuscript writing	
2. Berthold Koletzko	principal investigator and guarantor of the study, designed study protocol, contributed to writing of the manuscript	
3. Joana Hoyos	enrolment of subjects, conduct of study, acquisition and introduction of data, contribute to manuscript writing	Joana Hoyos
4. Marta Zaragoza-Jordana	acquisition and introduction of data, contribute to manuscript writing	
5. Anna Dobrzanska		

weitere Autoren bitte auf ein gesondertes Blatt

Kumulative Dissertation – Bestätigung   Stand: 27.04.2009

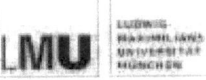 

Kumulative Dissertation

Bestätigung gem. § 4a Abs. 3 und 5 Promotionsordnung

Sonia A. Schiess
Doktorand/in

Einführung von Beikost in fünf europäischen Ländern
Titel der Dissertation

Hiermit bestätige ich, dass keiner der zur Promotion eingereichten Fachartikel Gegenstand einer anderen laufenden oder abgeschlossenen Dissertation ist.

Unterschrift Doktorand/in

Folgende **Ko-Autoren** bestätigen mit ihrer Unterschrift
- ihren Arbeitsanteil (Inhalt und Umfang) an den eingereichten Veröffentlichungen
- ihr Einverständnis zur Einreichung der Publikationen sowie,
- dass der jeweilige eingereichte Fachartikel nicht Gegenstand einer anderen laufenden oder abgeschlossenen Dissertation ist

Name Ko-Autor	Arbeitsanteil (Inhalt und Umfang)	Unterschrift Ko-Autor
1. Fiammetta Vecchi	enrolment of subjects, conduct of study, acquisition and introduction of data, contribute to manuscript writing	
2. Berthold Koletzko	principal investigator and guarantor of the study, designed study protocol, contributed to writing of the manuscript	
3. Jeanne Hoyos	enrolment of subjects, conduct of study, acquisition and introduction of data, contribute to manuscript writing	
4. Marta Zaragoza-Jordana	acquisition and introduction of data, contribute to manuscript writing	
5. Anna Dobrzanska		

weitere Autoren bitte auf ein gesondertes Blatt

Kumulative Dissertation_Bestätigung   Stand_27.04.2009

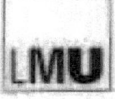 

Kumulative Dissertation

Bestätigung gem. § 4a Abs. 3 und 5 Promotionsordnung

Sonia A. Schiess

Doktorand

Einführung von Beikost in fünf europäischen Ländern

Titel der Dissertation

Hiermit bestätige ich, dass keiner der zur Promotion eingereichten Fachartikel Gegenstand einer anderen laufenden oder abgeschlossenen Dissertation ist.

Unterschrift Doktorand

Folgende Ko-Autoren bestätigen mit ihrer Unterschrift

- ihren Arbeitsanteil (Inhalt und Umfang) an den eingereichten Veröffentlichungen,
- ihr Einverständnis zur Einreichung der Publikationen sowie,
- dass der jeweilige eingereichte Fachartikel nicht Gegenstand einer anderen laufenden oder abgeschlossenen Dissertation ist.

Name Ko-Autor	Arbeitsanteil (Inhalt und Umfang)	Unterschrift Ko-Autor
1. Fiammetta Vecchi	enrolment of subjects, conduct of study, acquisition and introduction of data, contribute to manuscript writing	
2. Berthold Koletzko	principal investigator and guarantor of the study, designed study protocol, contributed to writing of the manuscript	
3. Ioana Hoyos	enrolment of subjects, conduct of study, acquisition and introduction of data, contribute to manuscript writing	
4. Marta Zaragozá-Jordana	acquisition and introduction of data, contribute to manuscript writing	
5. Anna Dobrzanska	enrolment of subjects, conduct of study, acquisition and introduction of data	

weitere Autoren bitte auf ein gesondertes Blatt

Kumulative Dissertation - Bestätigung   Stand: 27.04.2009

Beitrag der Doktorandin Sonia A. Schiess

- Rekrutierung der Teilnehmer in München.
- Betreuung von den Müttern/Eltern im Bezug auf die 3-Tage Wiegeprotokolle.
- Eingabe der 3-Tage Wiegeprotokolle für München und Nürnberg (ca. 1523 x 3-Tage Wiegeprotokolle).
- Besuch der verschiedenen Studienzentren (study visits) mit dem Ziel eine möglichst standardisierte Datensammlung und Dateneingabe zu gewährleisten (Entwicklung und Durchführung von Beispiel-Ernährungsprotokollen und ihre Auswertung).
- Entwicklung einer „Beikostliste" für die Datenauswertung über die verzehrten Nahrungsmittel (4186 Nahrungsmittel wurden in 29 mögliche Zutaten-Kategorien aufgeteilt). Mit Beihilfe der Kollegen für die Ausländische Produkte.
- Die Datenauswertung von ca. 10.000 3-Tages-Wiegeprotokolle erfolgte vorzugsweise mit SPSS und mit Excel.
- Literaturrecherche und Redaktion der vier Publikationen/Manuskripte.
- Teilnahme an den halbjährigen Studientreffen.

Publikationen and Präsentationen

Introduction of potentially allergenic foods in the infants diet during the first year of life in five European countries. Schiess, SA, Grote V, Scaglioni S, Luque V, Martin F, Stolarczyk A, Vechi F, and Koletzko B. Ann Nutr Metab 2011;58:109–117

Methodology for longitudinal assessment of nutrient intake and dietary habits in Early childhood in a transnational multicenter study. Verwied-Jorky S, Schiess S, Luque V, Grote V, Scaglioni S, Vecchi F, Martin F, Stolarczyk A, Koletzko B, for the European Childhood Obesity Project. J Pediatr Gastroenterol Nutr. 2011 Jan;52(1):96-102.

Kongress Milanopediatria November 2010, Vortrag: Introduction of complementary Feeding in five European countries (www.milanopediatria.it)

Frühkindliche Ernährung und späteres Adipositasrisiko. Hinweise auf frühe Metabolische Programmierung. Koletzko B, Schiess S, Brands B, Haile G, Demmelmair H, von Kries R, Grote V. Bundesgesundheitsblatt Gesundheitsfroschung Gesundheitsschutz 2010 Jul;53(7):666-73

Prävention der kindlichen Adipositas durch die Säuglingsernährung. Koletzko B, Grote V, Schiess S, Verwied-Jorky S, Brands B, Demmelmair H, von Kries R. Monatsschrift Kinderheilkunde 2010; 158: 553-563.

Beitrag Doktorandin

Introduction of complementary feeding in five European countries. Kongress The Power of Programming, München, 6.- 8.Mai 2010. Vortrag.

Intake of energy providing liquids during the first year of life in five European countries. Schiess SA, Grote V, Scaglioni S, Luque V, Martin F, Stolarczyk A, Vechi F, and Koletzko B. Clinical Nutrition 2010 (in press).

Solid introduction and growth in the first two years of life in formula-fed children. V.Grote, S.Schiess, B.Koletzko, for the European Childhood Obesity Trial Study Group. 6th World Congress DOHAD, Santiago de Chile, November 2009. Poster präsentation.

Introduction of complementary feeding in 5 European countries. S.Schiess, F.Confalionieri, V.Grote, J.Hoyos, V.Luque, F.Martin, G.Méndez, S.Scaglioni, A.Stolarczyk, F.Vecchi, A.Xhonneux, B.Koletzko. Nutrition and Nurture Conference, Grange-over-Sans, United Kingdom, September 2009. Vortrag.

Introduction of complementary feeding in five European countries. Schiess S, Grote V, Scaglioni S, Luque V, Martin F, Stolarczyk A, Vechi F, and Koletzko B. Journal of Pediatrics Gastroenterology and Nutrition 2009; 49, 1-8.

Beikosteinführung in fünf europäischen Ländern. S.Schiess, F.Confalionieri, V.Grote, J.Hoyos, V.Luque, F.Martin, G.Méndez, S.Scaglioni, A.Stolarczyk, F.Vecchi, A.Xhonneux, B.Koletzko. 104. Jahrestagung der Deutschen Gesellschaft für Kinder- und Jugendmedizin. Munich, Germany. September 2008. Vortrag.

Standard Operating Procedures to assess dietary intake in formula fed babies of the Childhood Obesity Programme (QLK1-2001-00389). Luque V, Mendez G, Closa R, Escribano J, Garcia-Closas R, Schiess S, Vecchi F, Hoyos J, Stolarczyk A, Koletzko B for the CHOP Study team. Early nutrition programming & health outcomes in later live: obesity & beyond. Pre-congres Satellite Meeting of 15th European Congress on Obesity. 20th -21th April 2007. Budapest (HUNGARY).

Elaboración de una herramienta para la valoración de la ingesta dietética en bebés alimentados con formula infantil. Méndez G., Luque V., Schiess S., Tedeschi S., Martin F., Stolarczyk A. III Congreso AEDN y I Congreso Luso Español de alimentación, nutrición y dietética. Madrid, Spain. Octubre 2006.

Estándares para la valoración de la ingesta dietética en bebés alimentados con lactancia artificial utilizados en el proyecto "EU Childhood Obesity: Early Programming by Infant Nutrition" (QLK1-2001-00389). Luque V., Méndez G., Schiess S., Vecchi F., Hoyos J., Stolarczyk A. III Congreso AEDN y I Congreso Luso Español de alimentación, nutrición y dietética. Madrid, Spain. Octubre 2006.

Protein intake in the first year of life: a risk factor for later obesity? The E.U. Childhood Obesity Project Koletzko B, Broekaert I, Demmelmair H, Franke J, Hannibal I, Oberle D, Schiess S, Baumann BT, Verwied-Jorky S; EU Childhood Obesity Project.. Adv Exp Med Biol 2005;569:69-79.

Is the crying behaviour in infants up to the age of 3 months influenced by the type of early feeding ? S.Schiess, D.Oberle, I.Broekaert, A.Reith, S.Verwied-Jorky, B.Koletzko. ESPGHAN Nutrition Summer School, Anavyssos, Greece. September 2005. Vortrag.

Is the crying behaviour in infants up to the age of 3 months influenced by the type of early nutrition ? S.Schiess, D.Oberle, I.Broekaert, A.Reith, S.Verwied-Jorky, B.Koletzko. World Congress of Paediatrics, Gastroenterology, Hepatology and Nutrition, in Paris, France. July 2004. Poster Präsentation.

Is the crying behaviour in infants up to the age of 3 months influenced by the type of early nutrition ? Is the crying behaviour in infants up to the age of 3 months influenced by the type of early nutrition ? S.Schiess, D.Oberle, I.Broekaert, A.Reith, S.Verwied-Jorky, B.Koletzko. Precongress Workshop. Early Nutrition and its later consequences: new opportunities, Paris, France. July 2004. Poster Präsentation.

Beeinflusst die Ernährung des Säuglings das Vorkommen der Dreimonatskolik ? S.Schiess, D.Oberle, I.Broekaert, A.Reith, S.Verwied-Jorky, B.Koletzko. Ernährung 2004, Munich, Germany. May 2004. Poster Präsentation.

Childhood Obesity-Programming by Infant Nutrition

Name des Kindes: _____ Schwangerschaft/ID-Nr.: OP-□□-□
Geburtsdatum des Kindes: Tag / Monat / Jahr

Alter des Kindes: 4 Wochen

Verzehrsprotokoll am Ende von Monat 1

Wann haben Sie dieses Protokoll ausgefüllt? _____ (Tag 1)
Tag / Monat / Jahr

Milchzubereitung & Milchverzehr

Uhrzeit	Art der Milch (Sorte, Handelsname)	Wasser (ml)	Pulver (Anzahl der Löffel)	Getränkesorte		Sonstige*		angebotene Menge (ml)	verzehrtes Volumen (ml)	Dauer der Ration (Minuten)
				Sorte, Handelsname	Anzahl der Löffel	Sorte, Handelsname	(g ml oder Löffel)			

*z.B.: B-Tee, Wasser, Säfte, Wasser + Zucker, Kamill-K.-Zuprofen, sonstiges

Sonstige Flüssigkeitsaufnahme

Uhrzeit	Art der Flüssigkeit (Sorte, Handelsname)	angebotene Menge (ml)	verzehrtes Volumen (ml)	Alter, wenn zum ersten Mal gegeben (Wochen)

Verzehr von fester Nahrung

Uhrzeit Mahlzeit	wo wurde die Mahlzeit eingenommen? (zu Hause, Orts...)	Angaben zu verzehrten Lebensmitteln (inkl. Zubereitungsart, Sorte, Eigenschaften, Handelsname)	angebotene Menge	nicht verzehrte Menge	Code (bitte nicht ausfüllen)

Beschreibung des Rezepts

Menge	Lebensmittel + Zutaten (inkl. Zubereitungsart)

Beschreibung des Rezepts

Menge	Lebensmittel + Zutaten (inkl. Zubereitungsart)

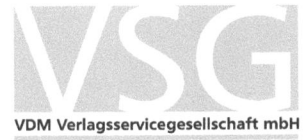

Die VDM Verlagsservicegesellschaft sucht für wissenschaftliche Verlage abgeschlossene und herausragende

Dissertationen, Habilitationen, Diplomarbeiten, Master Theses, Magisterarbeiten usw.

für die kostenlose Publikation als Fachbuch.

Sie verfügen über eine Arbeit, die hohen inhaltlichen und formalen Ansprüchen genügt, und haben Interesse an einer honorarvergüteten Publikation?

Dann senden Sie bitte erste Informationen über sich und Ihre Arbeit per Email an *info@vdm-vsg.de*.

Sie erhalten kurzfristig unser Feedback!

VDM Verlagsservicegesellschaft mbH
Dudweiler Landstr. 99
D - 66123 Saarbrücken

Telefon +49 681 3720 174
Fax   +49 681 3720 1749

www.vdm-vsg.de

Die VDM Verlagsservicegesellschaft mbH vertritt

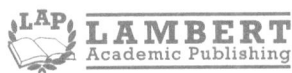
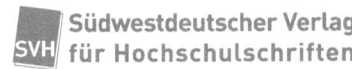

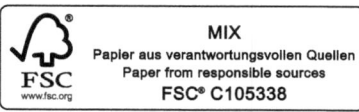

Printed by Books on Demand GmbH, Norderstedt / Germany